Incidental Finding

Essays on
Renal Cell Carcinoma

compiled and edited by
Cynthia Chauhan

Michael L. Blute, M.D.,
medical editor for professional content

Incidental Finding
Essays on
Renal Cell Carcinoma

Copyright © 2005
Cynthia Chauhan
Tallgrass Books—Wichita, Kansas
tallgrassbooks@aol.com

Library of Congress Control Number: 2005908046
ISBN Number: 0-9723827-1-2

Graphic Design & Book layout by Larry G. Nichols II
Printed in the U.S.A. by Mennonite Press, Inc., Newton, KS
First Printing December, 2005.
— Cover concept created by Cynthia Chauhan.
— Cover photographs courtesy Dr. Panos Z. Anastasiadis,
  Pamela Kreinest, and Dr. John A. Copland.

KNOWLEDGE IS POWER.

—Hobbes, Leviathan

This book is dedicated to

STEVE DUNN
1956–2005

*A fearless, tireless, brilliant advocate
for kidney cancer patients
who taught us the questions to ask,
and
gave us the courage to ask them.*

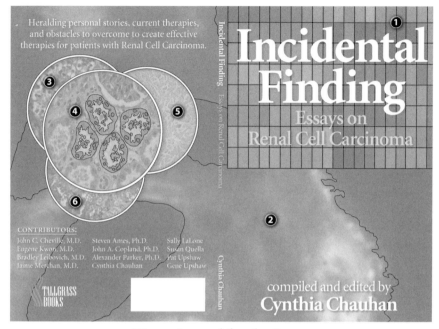

Figure Legend *for the* Cover

① Dendogram or heatmap representing expression levels of genes from patient-matched normal kidney and renal cell carcinoma (RCC) tissues. A new technology called genomics that examines all genes expressed in tissues allowing for identification of altered genes between normal and tumor tissues. For more see Chapter 5.

② Immunohistochemistry (IHC) technology used to identify protein expression in tissues and cells. This is a diagnostic tool that can be used to identify aberrant protein expression in tumor tissues as well as to determine whether a tumor may respond to a molecular targeted therapy.

③ Histological section of clear cell RCC stained with eosin and hematoxylin. The white area within the cell is the characteristic that distinguishes clear cell RCC from other subtypes of RCC. Clear cell RCC is the most common form of RCC. For more on the histology of RCC and occurrence, see Chapter 6.

④ Histological section of normal kidney tissue observed at a 40 fold magnification, under a light microscope. This allows visualization of cell structure and histological analysis of tissues leading to diagnosis for cancer. For more see Chapter 6. Tissue is stained with eosin and hematoxylin. Basophilic nuclei are stained "blue" with hematoxylin. Eosinophilic cytoplasm, connective, and all other tissues are counterstained "red" with eosin. Within the detailed areas are the proximal tubules from which one of the major subtypes of RCC arises.

⑤ Histological section of papillary RCC stained with eosin and hematoxylin. The finger-like structures or papillary are characteristic of this subtype of RCC. Papillary RCC is the second most common form of RCC.

⑥ Immunostaining (brown staining) of a protein identified by genomic profiling to be over expressed in clear cell RCC. The brown staining verifies that this protein is expressed.

PREFACE

One sunny spring afternoon, a dear friend and I were talking about the stormy world of renal cell carcinoma. We had just come from the kidney cancer support group meeting that I facilitate. We were both haunted not only by how little understood kidney cancer is by both lay and medical communities but also by how frustrating it is that people with renal cell carcinoma are too frequently told, in one way or another, to go home, enjoy what's left of their lives, and die.

It had been a day when three newly diagnosed stage IV renal cell patients had come to the group with many questions, great sadness, clear fear, overwhelming physical pain, and little awareness of options. They had been seen by oncologists but were completely lost. They knew they wanted to fight for their lives but they had no arsenals of knowledge or resources. They were desperate.

My friend looked at me in that deep way true friends have and said, "Cynthia, you have to write a book about this."

I laughed and said, "Oh, sure, just like that."

My friend persisted, "If not you, then who? You know that you can do this."

I thought about it and realized that I can write a book about renal cell carcinoma, that it makes no sense for me to wait for someone else to do it. So, I decided to write this book. Then I thought about what I want to convey and realized that the book I want to put out for public readership is a book of essays by professionals who work with renal cell carcinoma and by patients who live with renal cell carcinoma. I want to offer a glimpse for readers of the essence of our days, the struggles of patients to live, bolstered by the efforts of physicians and scientists to understand, treat, and work to cure renal cell carcinoma.

A question that you may ask is, "How did she choose her contributors?" The answer is simpler than you may suspect. I chose people whom I know and respect, people whom I believe have something worthwhile to say that needs to be available to a wide audience.

Whom do I know? I know physicians and researchers at the Mayo Clinic because that is where I receive my care. It is important to state that while my professional contributors all happen to practice at the Mayo Clinic, this is neither a Mayo Clinic publication nor a Mayo Clinic endorsed publication. It is a personal response to being diagnosed with a deadly, poorly understood cancer.

I know other patients with renal cell carcinoma because I facilitate a support group for kidney cancer patients and their caregivers, because I belong to a kidney cancer listserv, and because I go to meetings around the country for people with renal cell carcinoma. These patients receive their care at many different facilities. None of them know or are patients of the physicians contributing to this book. Their common bonds are that they have renal cell carcinoma and that they know me. They also do not know each other.

It really is that simple and straightforward. Invitation of all contributors is my personal choice based on my relationships with these extraordinary people. The professional contributors and patients do not know each other and neither group had any input into whose work I included in the book. That they are all included does not mean that any one contributor agrees with or would approve what another contributor says. It simply means that each of these remarkable people trusts me to not distort their contribution and to put out a book that attempts to speak the truth, even though that truth is sometimes neither pleasant nor hopeful. That everyone whom I asked to write agreed is a gift of uncommon, true charity to me and, I hope, to you.

If you know something about this disease and wonder, "Why didn't she include this or that world-famous renal cell carcinoma specialist?" The answer is that I don't have a special relationship with him or her and this book is a personal response to a death-dealing malignancy.

The renal cell carcinoma patients and their caregivers who contributed their stories were given the choice of anonymity. Cancer unalterably changes our lives but it is a very personal experience. I honor the courage of these wonderful people in choosing to share their identity as they open their experiences to public scrutiny. Each of them has made a decision to recapitulate a painful, uncertain journey in the hope of enlightening others about the horror of renal cell carcinoma. I am grateful for their courage and generous spirit.

The professional contributors gave freely and generously of their knowledge and understanding to make this book possible. I want to emphasize that they have given *freely*. No one of them receives any compensation for this work beyond the altruistic sensibility that they are educating people they may never meet to the devastating cancer called renal cell carcinoma. I have chosen not to do biographic sketches of the professional contributors but, if you are interested in their credentials, which are extensive, you will easily access them by googling their names on the web.

The order in which the authors' contributions appear in the book is arbitrary. I start with the urologist because that person is often a kidney cancer patient's first contact once kidney cancer is suspected. I continue with how I might like to learn about renal cell carcinoma if I were new to it, interspersing technical and patient chapters to accent each other. For ease of reading, all references are grouped in an appendix at the end of the book. I choose the chapter on immunotherapeutic approaches as the closing chapter because it is a beacon of hope to those of us diagnosed with renal cell carcinoma.

It is a good thing to hold onto hope. If you are a renal cell carcinoma patient and take only one message from this book, let that message be that there is hope and you have the right to seek the best care from specialists with particular expertise in renal cell carcinoma. Renal cell carcinoma is different from other cancers but it is not an automatic death sentence.

I also want to thank my friends, Rita Teller, Carol Ablah, and Guy MacDonald who read the manuscript for "reader friendliness" for me. They were not, before embarking on this labor of love, knowledgeable about kidney cancer. They brought fresh eyes to the reading to help assure the essays are accessible to people not immersed in the world of kidney cancer.

As always, working with the wonderful people at Mennonite Press is a gift in itself.

Incidental
Finding

INTRODUCTION

Rumi, the legendary Persian poet philosopher, tells this story:
> *The Sufi's pupil asked his elder, "How do you feel?"*
> *The Sufi replied, "Like one who has risen in the morning*
> *and does not know whether he will be dead in the evening."*
> *The pupil responded, "But that is the situation of all people."*
> *To which the wise Sufi replied, "Yes, but how many of them feel it?"*

My answer to the Sufi would be, "Those of us who live with cancer. We understand and know well that we may be dead by evening."

Saturday evenings of my childhood, we bumped down that red dirt country road named after the money General Lee was said to have buried there. Beginning to smell Tante Lucille's biscuits before the turn for her house, eager to be hugged and kissed silly by her nine kids, my sister and I chorused, "Are we there yet?"

We always ate crusty baguettes at home. Hot, soft biscuits as big as plates and as light as cotton balls were Tante Lucille's treat. When our stomachs were full of flaky biscuits drenched in fresh churned butter, we'd sit out back under the stars, drink sweet tea, and listen to Henri and Beau pick their guitars and sing about love gone wrong. We didn't know we were building memories. We were just kids passing time while Mama and Tante Lucille visited.

Nunc Pierre was a good-hearted trickster, a trapper completely at home in the swamps of south Louisiana. Following his prey, he moved his family around the wetlands. I remember the house in the swamps of Slidell. We had to drive around a bayou on a road that was more imaginative use of ruts than road. At the end were stacks of cages holding various sizes of alligators. Racks of muskrat pelts leaned against the house. Fearless children of every size poured helter-skelter out the door and ran alongside the car as we lurched around the bayou. They grabbed us and hugged us silly, whirling us around, tumbling with us on the dirt driveway, all of us laughing with the pure joy of being alive and together. Exhausted by delight, we laid sprawled all over each other in the dirt. Then we laughed some more just because.

Inside, standing at the stove was sweet Tante Lucille, unruffled by all of life's demands and surprises. Her calmness wrapped itself around her rambunctious children and restless husband in a cloud of love.

It is this everydayness of relationships which gives meaning and depth to my life. It is the people whom I love and who love me who give me reason to continue when life seems too overwhelming, when I can't imagine having to face one more devastating health problem. Then, I remember someone I love or am touched by someone's caring and it is all not only worthwhile but also a gift.

As a little girl, I would sometimes go to work with my daddy. I'd stand rubbing my sleepy eyes while Mama dressed me in a starched pinafore and plaited my long blonde hair. Then Daddy and I would cross Lake Pontchartrain in the predawn pitch to dawning adventure. Once in New Orleans, Daddy strolled while I skipped and danced down Decatur Street to Morning Call for breakfast coffee and beignets before he would start work. Small moments with other people fill my heart with the gift of life-sustaining memories.

Each moment of life is a gift of unique beauty. Sometimes the gift is evident; sometimes it is wrapped in weird paper. Cancer is the weirdest paper that has ever wrapped gifts to me. Ugly, terrifying kidney cancer wrapped itself around beautiful gifts unimaginable to me before I received them. There are about 200,000 of us in the United States living with kidney cancer at any given moment with about 32,000 new cases and 12,000 deaths each year. Tracking from the mid 1970s to now indicates the incidence is increasing at a rate of about 2.5% per year. One half of all people diagnosed with renal cell carcinoma have or will develop metastatic disease. Funding and public knowledge are not keeping pace with the disease. Statistics are impersonal, cancer is not. It is a very personal, unexpected experience.

Through having kidney cancer, I not only have reframed my life but also have met extraordinary people who face this devastating disease with courage and grace. I have also discovered exemplary professionals who dedicate themselves with unbending determination to providing and finding effective treatments and eventually a cure for those of us with kidney cancer in all of its pernicious forms.

This book is a tribute to those people. It is also an invitation to those of you lucky enough not to be touched by kidney cancer to glimpse our world. We offer you a collection of the experiences of kidney cancer patients interspersed with the perspectives of the professionals who work diligently on our behalf. For some, reading this will be a reminder of your own journey. For others, it will be an exploration of uncharted country. For all who turn these pages, we seek to offer understanding, to kindle hope.

Incidental
Finding

TABLE *of* CONTENTS

CHAPTER 1

The Urologist's Role *in the* Treatment *of* Renal Cell Carcinoma
by Bradley Leibovich, M.D.

I'm going to start out by telling you a little bit about why I went into urology. I initially wanted to be a family practice physician but eventually found that I liked surgery and decided to go into surgical oncology of some sort. When I found out that urologists could reliably cure people with surgery without need for additional treatment and that the negative impact on quality of life from urologic surgery was minimal, it immediately appealed to me as a potentially very gratifying specialty. This is inconceivable to many people who don't understand what urology is or what urologic oncologists do. I've been asked multiple times questions like, "What is it like to be a 'urinologist'?" That is, people, thinking that I study urine all day long, ask if it's boring to study urine all day long. It's certainly not a field than anyone goes into for having interesting conversations around the dinner table or for trying to be impressive. However, I don't know of any other surgical field that is as gratifying. It is unique because not only do you get to care for your patients medically, but also you need to have a good understanding of renal and smooth muscle physiology, as well as of the unique and fascinating biology of urologic malignancies including prostate cancer, bladder cancer, kidney cancer, and testicular cancer.

That is how I came to this engrossing profession. I am going to frame information about the urologist's role in kidney cancer as case presentations. I think this is a readily meaningful and useful method for me to give you very specific information about surgical treatments for renal cell carcinoma. I will caution you that these are not all success stories. It is a sad, sad truth that some of my patients die in spite of my best efforts. That is the reality of renal cell carcinoma.

The first patient is a young 38 year old woman who had sought care for a chronic cough and right side flank pain. At the time of referral to me, she had already had a chest x ray and a CT scan without x ray dye because it was suspected the flank pain was due to kidney stones. Her cough was discovered to be an upper respiratory illness. No evidence of stones was seen on the CT scan. However, the contour of the kidney on the left side was a little unusual. A subsequent CT scan was done with contrast. This revealed a small, approximately 2½ cm. (about an inch) large tumor deep within the substance of the kidney, barely altering the contour of the surface of the kidney. It was located in the area of the hilum where the blood vessels enter and exit the kidney. She had been told that this was definitely a cancer. That was about all of the information that she had gotten before being referred to me.

At our first meeting, she and I had a lengthy conversation in which I went over her blood tests, her urine tests, her CT scan of the belly, her chest x ray. My secretary had already ordered a CT scan of the chest which is what we normally do to complete the staging for kidney cancer. If someone has a suspected kidney cancer, we are concerned about the potential areas of spread. The most common are the lungs, the lymph nodes, the bone, the liver, and the brain. If we narrow those down to ones that are common, the lymph nodes and the lungs, those are seen very readily on CT scan. Spread to the bone is very uncommon without bone pain so for small kidney tumors we usually don't get a bone scan. Spread to the brain or the spinal cord without symptoms is extremely uncommon and is also very uncommon with a small renal mass. We had a lengthy discussion about her prognosis which was, of course, excellent.

I explained to her that a lesion of this size has at least a one in five chance of being a benign tumor, which is not a cancer. Benign tumors in the kidney are very common, especially with the smaller tumors. I also explained that our data would indicate that a smaller tumor, if it is a cancer, is very likely to be a non-aggressive variety of kidney cancer. We then discussed the potential surgical options and non-surgical options, including doing nothing and simply observing which is certainly a reasonable approach for someone older than she. However, at this young age, I recommended against simple observation.

We discussed the fact that a biopsy of the lesion is often not helpful because biopsies are inaccurate for kidney cancer. Kidney cancers are frequently very heterogeneous or inhomogeneous. Therefore, if the biopsy is done in one area, it may look like a cancer but in another area, it may look benign. This makes it very difficult for the pathologist to give us a reliable reading.

We discussed non-surgical options including ablative technologies in which the urologist, working in conjunction with an interventional radiologist, sticks a needle into the tumor through the skin using imaging guidance, either an ultrasound CT scan or an MRI. The tumor is then either frozen with cryosurgery or heated, usually with radiofrequency. I recommended against this also for her at this young age because we do not have extended follow-up on these technologies and I am not sure that the long-term cure rates will be as good as are achieved with surgical removal. We also discussed the fact that this would not help us in getting an accurate pathological diagnosis which is important for someone in this age group when we have to worry about her long-term surveillance.

In the end, I recommended that her tumor be surgically removed which options included laparoscopic or open approaches. I explained to her that, with the small size of the tumor, we would always favor doing a partial nephrectomy due to the chance that this is either a benign lesion or a non-aggressive kidney cancer. I also explained to her that the location of the tumor would make a laparoscopic partial nephrectomy extremely difficult. It is more difficult to control bleeding with a laparoscopic approach than it is with an open approach. Laparoscopy is currently reserved for tumors that are located more peripherally on the kidney rather than deep within the center of the kidney as hers was located.

We discussed the pros and cons of a partial nephrectomy versus a radical nephrectomy and I explained to her the data on partial nephrectomy providing a better quality of life, a better psychological outcome according to some studies, as well as being equivalent to a radical nephrectomy to cure cancer with a lower likelihood of problems with kidney function down the road. Given that information, she said that she was in favor of the partial nephrectomy approach.

We talked about how the surgery would be performed with a flank incision and the steps involved in the surgery as well as the risks. The main risks include bleeding, loss of the kidney, urine leak, as well as the standard other problems that can happen with any surgery. It is possible to leak urine from the site because cutting across the collecting system can result in a weakness in the side of the kidney that allows urine to leak out of the kidney rather than go down the ureter.

For surgery, she was positioned on the table on her side and the incision was made around the twelfth rib on her side. The kidney was exposed and we removed the surrounding fat from around the entire kidney. The kidney was inspected to make sure there was no other area of tumor. This was relatively straightforward in her case because despite the fact that the majority of the tumor was within the kidney, it did distort the contour of the kidney, making it easy to see where the lesion was located.

Combining that with what I could see on the CT scan allowed me to very accurately remove the kidney tumor along with some normal surrounding kidney tissue. The pathologist immediately indicated that the margin or the edge of the specimen was clean of cancer and that the main specimen itself was a grade 1 papillary renal cell carcinoma. The defect or the hole in the kidney was closed surgically by sewing it back together, providing compression to prevent bleeding. At the end of her closure, she had lost very little blood and the incision appeared to be watertight. A drain was left in place. She was transferred to the recovery room.

I spoke with her husband, explaining to him that everything went extremely well and that she was highly likely to be cured of her kidney cancer. After a three-day hospital stay, she left the hospital feeling well, taking a minimal dose of a narcotic for pain. The incision on her side, which measures eight to ten cm (3½ to 4 inches), has healed nicely. To date, her kidney function remains completely unchanged from her preoperative levels. Over three years after the surgery, she has no evidence of recurrence, is doing well, and has required no other treatment. I continue to see her for regular follow-up.

The next patient is a 45 year old man who was having a routine physical. His physician noticed that he had a microscopic amount of blood in his urine. Microscopic amounts of blood in the urine are a potential sign of a problem with the kidneys, the ureters, or the bladder. The main concerns when we have findings of blood in the urine, either visible or microscopic, are tumors or stones, but there are other potential problems as well such as cysts, problems with abnormal bleeding, trauma, and medical conditions that affect the kidneys. The standard evaluation for blood in the urine has now become an evaluation with an imaging study. In the past this was an IVP or urogram. This has been replaced essentially by CT scanning technology. This patient had a CT urogram which is a CT scan that looks at the drainage system of the kidneys as well as the meat of the kidneys. He was noted to have a tumor in the left kidney. It was approximately six cm (2 inches) in size, located in the center of the kidney in the area where it could have been a tumor of the collecting system, that is the lining of the kidney, or the parenchyma of the kidney.

The patient had a history of smoking as well and smoking increases the risk of renal cell carcinoma by a factor of approximately two. However, it increases the risk of urothelial carcinoma, or cancer of the lining of the kidney, the ureters, and the bladder by a factor of twenty. So, it was important to complete his evaluation and ascertain whether this was a tumor of the lining of the kidney versus a tumor of the meat of the kidney. We also wanted to be sure we weren't missing anything else. As far as I could tell from the CT scan and urogram, the lining of the kidney looked okay. However, it was vital to make certain and to check the bladder.

The patient and I discussed the possibility that this was a tumor of the meat of the kidney versus a tumor of the lining. I explained to him the risk associated with smoking. Thankfully, he had already quit smoking. We decided to investigate him with a cystoscopy which is a procedure where you look inside the bladder with a flexible scope. It takes approximately two to five minutes, is done in the clinic setting, and remarkably causes minimal pain with the patient awake using a local anesthetic in the urethra. I also explained to him that at the time of the cystoscopy, we would collect some of his urine, looking for cancerous cells within the urine which is common when people have urethelial carcinoma. We would also inject some x ray dye backwards up to his left kidney to help us to get a better idea of where the tumor was located. The cystoscopy as well as the retrograde pyelogram, which is the injection of x ray dye backwards up into the kidney were both completely unremarkable and looked entirely normal. The urine came back without evidence of cancer cells in the urine. He had had a chest CT scan ordered which was clean. The remainder of his laboratory tests were all perfectly normal.

I reviewed his laboratory test results with him. We discussed the options for treating this. Because of the location of the tumor, I did not think that a partial nephrectomy was feasible as the tumor was located where the main artery that enters the kidney spreads out throughout the kidney and I was relatively certain that this would result in destroying his kidney in the process of trying to remove the tumor. I explained to him that we thought that this was a tumor of the meat of the kidney which is an important consideration because renal parenchymal tumor or renal cell carcinoma does not respond to chemotherapy or radiation. Our primary mode of treatment of renal cell carcinoma is surgical removal prior to the tumor's spreading. I reviewed with him the fact that urothelial carcinoma is an entirely different sort of tumor which does often respond to chemotherapy and this strongly alters how it is managed.

We reviewed the films in detail and I explained to him the process for removing his kidney and some lymph nodes adjacent to the kidney which appeared to be normal based on the scans. We discussed the options of open radical nephrectomy versus a laparoscopic radical nephrectomy.

I explained to him that with a qualified laparoscopic surgeon who could do regional lymph node removal he would likely have a very short stay in the hospital, minimal pain, and a very rapid recovery. These are certainly major advantages over the open surgical technique. He was enamored with this. He went to one of my colleagues with particular expertise in laparoscopic technique. My colleague performed a hand-assisted laparoscopic partial nephrectomy through a small, 6 mm, incision in the lower abdomen, below the umbilicus. Through this incision, the surgeon placed his hand into the belly. At the same time, he used two tiny 5 mm. to 10 mm. long incisions for access with the scopes. The surgeon removed the tumor within about an hour and ten minutes. The blood loss was extremely minimal. The patient was in the hospital only one night and went home on Tylenol only. His tumor was confined to the kidney. The lymph nodes that were removed were clear of tumor. He had a grade 2 clear cell renal cell carcinoma. It was extremely likely to be cured. He has not yet come back to me for follow up but the surgeon tells me that this patient is doing very well and is back to all of his normal activities only about a month later.

The next patient is a 68 year old man with no family history of any malignancies and no personal history of any problems who self-referred to me for a second opinion. He was told by his local surgeon that he needed to have both kidneys removed and to go on dialysis. He had a CT scan of the belly obtained for diffuse abdominal pain which is likely due to irritable bowel syndrome and completely unrelated to his renal masses. However, the scan did show a mass within each kidney. He had a mass taking over approximately ½ of his right kidney and ⅓ of the left kidney. The masses appeared solid and well-circumscribed. I said that his tumors were not likely to be the cause of his pain because the area around the kidney can become quite full of an extremely large tumor prior to a person feeling pain.

It is very common for people to show up with very large tumors that are asymptomatic. Unfortunately, this is one of the reasons that about ⅓ of the renal cell carcinoma cases do not show any signs or symptoms until after the tumor has metastasized. I showed him his films. He had had a CT scan of the chest, a blood test, and a urine test done by us. He had brought with him CT scans of the abdomen and pelvis. I explained to him that an alternative was to try to do a partial nephrectomy on each kidney or a radical nephrectomy on one side and a partial nephrectomy on the other side in the hopes that we would salvage enough kidney tissue that he would not require dialysis. Hemodialysis is usually done three days per week and during the days of dialysis the patient is hooked up to the machine for a few hours. In general, most people would find quality of life superior with some kidney function and off of dialysis. He was well aware of this and wanted to avoid dialysis at all costs. He was interested in the possibility of nephron-sparing approach. I explained to him that with the size of these tumors and with their appearance on scan, I was relatively comfortable that these were renal cell carcinomas and we discussed all of the potential problems we could encounter.

I explained that we could go through the flank, that is, the side, for each kidney and do it together in one operation or stage two operations or we could make an incision underneath the ribcage in the front which is a chevron incision that is shaped like an upside-down "v" on the front of the belly. The main advantages of this are the better access to the great vessels, which are the aorta and the vena cava; the ability to do a more extended lymph node dissection; and the ability to access both kidneys through the same incision. The main disadvantages are that it is a much larger incision and it is probably more painful. When we come through the front we have to move the intestines out of the way to get to the kidneys which are in the back of the belly. This results in what is called an ileus in which the intestines don't work for several days meaning that he can't eat or drink and is in the hospital longer than with the flank approach which is usually only a two or three day hospital stay. The transabdominal or transperoneal approach can have up to a week's stay.

We discussed the disadvantages of partial nephrectomy including the higher risk of bleeding, although significant bleeding that is life-threatening would be unlikely. I did explain that he would need blood transfusions. We discussed the possibility that, despite the fact that we are trying to save his kidneys, he may wind up with inadequate kidney function and need dialysis anyway. We discussed the possibility of a urine leak and that this is usually fixed by simply placing some additional tubes after which the leaks usually heal on their own. We discussed the possibility of tumor recurrence within the kidney which, based on our data, is about six percent of kidneys which had partial nephrectomies. We discussed the possibility of cure which is similar for partial nephrectomy and radical nephrectomy. That is, the likelihood of dying appears to be the same for partial nephrectomy or radical nephrectomy. However, the possibility of having a recurrence that would need treatment is higher for a partial nephrectomy since, obviously, there is no chance for a recurrence in the same kidney with a radical nephrectomy. We discussed the remainder of potential problems, things like heart attack, stroke, blood clots, blood clots which travel to the lungs which are called pulmonary emboli. We discussed the possibility of death from the surgery, infections, and the remainder of potential complications at length. He indicated that he understood all of them, that he did want to be extremely aggressive but to maintain his kidneys and be off of dialysis if at all possible. We therefore agreed to proceed with a single operation, approaching both kidneys simultaneously through the front of the belly.

He went to the operating room, the chevron incision was made, and his abdomen was explored. I inspected the liver, gall bladder, pancreas, spleen, and stomach; felt both kidneys; and examined the intestines. There was no evidence of spread and the lymph nodes along the aorta and vena cava were not palpably enlarged.

I approached the larger tumor first. The artery to the kidney was dissected free, taking care not to manipulate the artery very much. The vein to the kidney was dissected free. A plastic bag was placed in the area surrounding the kidney. The anesthesiologist gave the patient intravenous Lasix and Mannitol to protect the kidney and the artery to the kidney was clamped. The kidney was cooled by packing it in ice. Once the kidney was completely cooled, the ice slush was removed from around the kidney and the tumor, which was in the lower portion of the kidney, was removed with a healthy rim of normal tissue. This resulted in approximately ½ of the kidney being removed. Because the artery was clamped, there was minimal bleeding. However, there was a large hole in the collecting system, the drainage system of the kidney, which was obvious and had to be closed with suture. I closed this and all individual arteries were sewn shut with small, absorbable sutures. The edges of the kidney were tied together with a special technique to compress the edges of the kidney and the clamp was released from the artery. The bleeding was very well controlled. There was no evidence of bleeding or leak from the kidney. The total amount of time that the artery was clamped was only eighteen minutes.

We then approached the opposite side. Because I had clamped the artery previously, I decided not to clamp the artery on this side. However, I did dissect it free so that I could clamp it if bleeding was encountered. This tumor was smaller. With a simple manual compression of the edges of the kidney and without clamping the artery, I was able to dissect this tumor free with a healthy rim of normal tissue surrounding it. The kidney was closed in a similar fashion. There was a smaller hole in the collecting system on this side that was also closed in a similar fashion. The patient lost minimal blood from this side. I then proceeded to remove all of the lymph nodes from around the arteries and veins that drain the kidneys and the main arteries that run up and down the back, the aorta and the vena cava.

The pathologist indicated that the margins on both of the tumors were clear. The larger tumor was a grade 3 clear cell renal cell carcinoma. The smaller tumor was an oncocytoma which is a benign tumor. All of the lymph nodes were free of cancer and normal. The patient had a post-operative creatinine of 1.8 which rose over the next few days to a peak of 2.7 which subsequently came down and settled around 2.

I have followed this patient for approximately four years now since the surgery. During this time he has had an excellent quality of life with stable kidney function. He has had a small recurrence in one kidney. Following an indeterminate biopsy, the lesion was treated with and completely destroyed by radiofrequency ablation. He has no evidence of metastatic spread and no evidence of further recurrences.

The next patient is an exception to the rule. This is a situation where we could tell prior to surgery exactly what we were dealing with. This is a young 28 year old woman who presented to her ob-gyn with severe right-sided flank pain. She had developed severe pain, lightheadedness, dizziness. When she arrived in the emergency room, her blood pressure, blood counts, and hemoglobin were noted to be low. A CT scan showed a tumor in the right kidney with bleeding around it. The two reasons this is an exception are that it was seen on the CT scan that some of the tumor had fat density—this is seen only with a tumor called an angiomyolipoma which is known to be a benign tumor that contains fat within it. Additionally, it is known that myolipomas can grow rapidly with fertility treatments or pregnancy. So the picture fit for the patient to have angiomyolipoma: It was a large tumor that had blood and it was not well-seen with the CT scan at the time of the bleed. We, therefore, allowed the patient to be stabled by her primary physicians.

She came back to see me in the clinic approximately six weeks later with a high-quality MRI which showed a tumor located dead center of the drainage center of the kidney with four renal arteries splayed around the tumor as opposed to the more common single renal artery. The tumor was obviously adjacent to the drainage system of the kidney and emarcated well within the center of the kidney. I discussed with the patient the options which included a radical nephrectomy and a partial nephrectomy. I explained that a partial nephrectomy would be technically very difficult due to the size and location of the tumor but that a radical nephrectomy seemed to be unnecessarily aggressive for a tumor that seemed very likely to be a benign angiomyolipoma. Therefore, she elected to proceed with a partial nephrectomy.

As this would be a complex surgery, I elected to approach this through a subcausal incision, which is an incision through the front of her belly underneath the rib cage on the right side. After moving the intestines out of the way and exposing the mass, it was apparent that the mass was adherent to the renal pelvis, or the major portion of the collecting system of the kidney. In addition, the four renal arteries were visible and one renal artery appeared to go right through the tumor. This renal artery was sacrificed and the tumor was meticulously removed from the center of the kidney taking care to preserve all of the blood vessels. Since we were not concerned that this was a cancer, it was quite a bit simpler to stay right on the edge of the tumor and not worry about removing some normal kidney tissue with it to assure a negative or clean margin. The tumor was dissected free and was peeled off of the collecting system and the renal pelvis. A small hole was made in the renal pelvis which was significantly thinned. I therefore extended the hole and placed a stent, a small thin plastic tube, which coiled up in the kidney and coiled in the bladder. We left the stent in place for six weeks after the surgery. The tumor was completely removed and the kidney survived with minimal negative impact to the kidney from removing one of the four renal arteries. This young patient did exceptionally well after the surgery, leaving the hospital after four days. Pathology confirmed that the tumor was a benign angiomyolipoma. Close follow up has revealed no evidence of recurrence and she has resumed her normal activities.

I saw the next two patients within a week of each other. The first one is a 48 year old man who also had blood in his urine. He came to us from elsewhere with a complete evaluation including all of the necessary blood tests, urine tests, a bone scan, CT scans of the chest, abdomen, and pelvis which revealed multiple nodules within the lungs which were clearly areas of metastatic spread, a large tumor in the left kidney measuring about 16 cm (about 6½ inches) in diameter, growing through the renal vein into the inferior vena cava, the big vein that runs up and down the back, up to just below the liver. We call this a renal vein and inferior vena cava tumor thrombus because this is actual tumor that has grown from the kidney through the vein into the vena cava. He also had a large lesion within the right lobe of the liver measuring approximately 4 cm (1¼ inch). Everything else looked completely normal.

I had a very lengthy discussion with this patient regarding the fact that, in general, we like to find kidney cancer before it has spread because there is no very effective systemic treatment for kidney cancer when it has spread. We discussed the benefit of aggressive surgical resection of as much tumor as can be removed followed by treatment with immunotherapy. I explained to him that there is lots of evidence that the immune system is meant to prevent us from getting cancer by removing abnormal cells from the body before they can grow into a cancer. We are beginning to understand the mechanisms that allow a cancer to grow and to escape the immune system. I explained that kidney cancer has had multiple instances over the years of areas of spread going away without active treatment. This occurs in about one out of 200 patients and is usually seen in pulmonary nodules, as this patient had, after removing the kidney that has the tumor in it. I explained that because of this evidence of the activity of the immune system which we presume is the principle reason for these tumors to go away, people have exploited the use of drugs that can enhance the immune system. I explained that the main two treatments are Interferon and Interleukin 2. The side effects of treatment are, in general, flu-like symptoms. However, the symptoms from high-dose Interleukin 2 treatment can be extremely severe. I discussed what our surgery would involve to remove the kidney tumor. I had the patient meet with one of our general surgeons who specializes in liver surgery to discuss the possibility of removing the liver tumor. He also met with a thoracic surgeon who thought that the nodules on the lungs were scattered too far throughout the lungs and were not surgically removable. The general surgeon, however, thought that with a partial resection of a portion of the right liver, the liver tumor could be removed. I explained to the patient that, even if we chose not to treat him aggressively for the areas of spread of his cancer, the tumor that has already gone up the vena cava would likely progress rapidly to his heart and cause his death very soon if we did not do something surgically. Considering that the patient had essentially no symptoms and was feeling very well, he elected to be aggressive with his treatment.

He underwent surgery through a trans-abdominal sub costal or chevron incision. I first moved the bowel from the left side of the belly towards the right and completely exposed the aorta, found the artery to the right kidney and tied that artery off. The kidney was mobilized on the left hand side inferiorly. Superiorly, the adrenal gland was intentionally dissected free from the kidney and left behind. This was because there was no involvement of the adrenal gland seen on the imaging and the patient could still have metastatic spread to the adrenal gland on the other side. If this happened, and I removed his left adrenal gland, he could wind up needing steroids because of lack of adrenal glands. If we had to give him steroids, that would raise the possibility that immunotherapy would be less effective. So, the left adrenal gland was left behind. Once the kidney had been mobilized, I started to dissect the left renal vein clear, which was quite distended with tumor thrombus. I was extremely careful not to manipulate this any more than necessary as it is quite possible for these tumor thrombi to break loose and travel to the lungs causing immediate death. Once this had been freed up, I then had to move the intestines from the right hand side over to expose the vena cava all the way up to the liver. A clamp was placed across the vena cava above the tumor thrombus which could be palpated in the vena cava. A clamp was placed across the right renal vein and a clamp was placed across the vena cava below the renal veins. The tumor was removed from the vena cava and the left renal vein was taken off of the vena cava. The vena cava was then closed. The tumor and the renal vein were wrapped and encased in surgical towels. The bowel was transposed back to the other side. The kidney with the tumor and the tumor thrombus were completely removed as well as all of the lymph nodes. The general surgeon came in and removed the right liver lesion. The left kidney tumor, the thrombus, and the liver lesion were all found to be grade 3 clear cell renal cell carcinoma. His lymph nodes were clean.

This patient had a very rough stay in the hospital. He developed hemoptosis which is coughing up blood. This was quite problematic. He had to have two procedures where the pulmonary physicians placed a scope into his lungs to cauterize bleeding points. This finally controlled the bleeding. However, a CT scan showed fairly rapid progression of his pulmonary disease. Despite this, he was able to get out of the hospital in two weeks feeling relatively well.

I discussed with him all of the potential options for treatment of his pulmonary nodules. Previously, he had already decided that he would travel to a facility closer to home to receive high-dose IL 2 treatment. He did this. High dose IL 2 is given as an inpatient procedure usually done with an infusion every eight hours for five days followed by a week to ten days out of the hospital, five days back in the hospital for infusion every eight hours and then a six to eight week rest period outside of the hospital at which point he returns to the hospital and repeats the process for five days in, seven to ten days out, five days in. At that point the treatments are complete. Potential complications of the treatment include drops in blood pressure, problems with kidney function, problems with the heart and lungs. Patients have to be monitored throughout the treatment for all of these complications. Patients also frequently get a severe flu-like syndrome which makes them feel quite miserable during the treatment.

This patient did, however, tolerate the treatment extremely well. Over the next several months he had serial scans which eventually showed that his disease within the lungs completely resolved without any evidence of disease visible in the lungs. His abdominal scans also showed no evidence of disease in the abdomen. His liver and kidney function were essentially normal and, once fully recovered from immunotherapy, he had no side effects from his treatment and led a perfectly normal life. Subsequently, he was found to have a brain lesion that was resected by one of our neurosurgeons and found to be kidney cancer. This was followed by whole brain radiation. The patient has done extremely well. He is now almost a year out from his brain metastasis resection and is still doing well without any evidence of disease. He has no residual neurological problems from the brain metastasis resection. He just recently sent me an email stating that he and his family are doing very well.

The second patient who came in that same week with a very similar story was a young man in his mid 50s with a persistent cough. Chest X rays showed nodules on the lungs. A CT scan of the chest also showed lung nodules and, at the bottom of the scan, showed, on his right kidney, a large tumor which grew up the vena cava to just above the liver. However, it was still within the abdomen. His evaluation included blood tests, urine tests, a chest CT scan, CT scans of the abdomen and pelvis. He had no other symptoms of his disease. He and I had in-depth discussions regarding the options. He also wanted to be very aggressive and proceed with surgery. His pulmonary nodules were not resectable but his kidney tumor and his vena cava thrombus were.

The patient was taken to the operating room. It was a simpler operation despite the fact that the thrombus went higher in the vena cava. It is always easier to operate on a right-sided tumor with a tumor thrombus than on a left-sided tumor with a tumor thrombus because the bowel doesn't have to be flipped back and forth. Incidentally, right-sided tumors are slightly more common than left-sided. His operation went well. He also had a grade 3 clear cell renal cell carcinoma. His post-operative recovery was completely uneventful. He left the hospital after five days, feeling remarkably well. We had arranged an appointment for him to come back and discuss starting immunotherapy a month after his surgery.

However, approximately three weeks after his discharge, he was brought into the emergency room by one of his family members who thought he was having a stroke. In fact, what he had was a large area of metastasis to the brain. The neurosurgeons thought this area was not resectable.   It was too large to be treated by gamma knife so he underwent radiation to the brain metastasis and whole brain radiation. With radiation and steroid therapy, all of his symptoms resolved. Unfortunately, all of the symptoms returned. He developed further metastases in the brain. His pulmonary metastases spread exceedingly rapidly, perhaps due to the steroids, perhaps just due to aggressive disease. Due to his rapid decline, he was never able to start immunotherapy and passed away within three months of his surgery.

It is remarkable to me that these two men came to me so closely together. Neither one of these men had sarcomatoid features in their specimens, neither of them had histologic tumor necrosis. Based on our predictive algorithms, the outcomes should have been different. The first patient should have done poorly and the second patient should have done well. This is why I do not like to use statistics when I talk with patients. I always explain to them that statistics are only good for papers and large groups of people. They are not good for predicting what will happen to one specific individual. If someone asks me what their chances are, I truthfully respond, "Well, someone's got to be a hundred percent and I'm always expecting that's going to be you."

The next patient is a 60 year old man two years away from retirement. Six years prior, he had had his right kidney removed for kidney cancer. He was followed up elsewhere for a few years and then told he didn't need follow-up anymore because he was cured. The first problem was that this man's entire kidney had been removed for a relatively small (3 cm or less than 1 inch) peripheral tumor, grade 2 clear cell renal cell carcinoma, for which I certainly would have advocated a partial rather than radical nephrectomy. The second problem was that he was told that he didn't need any follow-up at all and now, six years later, he has multiple tumors in his solitary kidney. This gentleman was extremely anxious and emotional. All that he wanted was to get through the end of his career and retire without having to go on disability.

We discussed the implications if his tumors riddling his kidney were kidney cancer, there was likelihood that he would lose his kidney. We discussed the options of simply proceeding to a radical nephrectomy which meant that he would be on dialysis for at least one to two years before anyone would consider giving him a kidney transplant. This is because, when you do a kidney transplant, you have to immunosuppress the patient. When you immunosuppress the patient, if there is any residual cancer anywhere, it will blossom and grow rapidly during the immunosuppression. Traditionally, the waiting period before someone would be considered an acceptable candidate for a transplant has been two years. More recently, if people have very good prognosis, that interval may be shortened, particularly if there is a living related donor available.

The patient did not like this option. He really wanted to make sure that he could finish his career without having to go on disability. We talked about partial nephrectomy or multiple enucleations of his tumors. He elected to do this. So, through the flank approach, I exposed the entire kidney and removed eight tumors from his kidney in one setting. Due to the fact that some tumors were very deep within the kidney and difficult to locate, we used intraoperative ultrasound to help localize the intrarenal tumors. After the eight tumors were removed, there was still one tumor deep within the kidney that appeared to be in a bad location. Therefore, intraoperatively, we used ultrasound guidance to place a radiofrequency probe into that lesion and ablated it. He had eight tumors removed and one tumor ablated with radiofrequency. The pathology on the eight tumors which were removed included five grade 2 clear cell renal cell carcinomas and three oncocytomas.

He has been coming back to see me every three months. He is extremely grateful to still have his kidney but he is still extremely anxious at each follow-up visit. He paces the room until I come in and doesn't want to know or discuss anything until I give him the results of his MRI. We follow him with MRIs because he does have chronic renal insufficiency although his creatinine has remained between 1.7 and 2.1. The MRIs over the past few years have shown multiple recurrences within that kidney which have been treated with percutaneous radiofrequency ablation or cryosurgery. We have biopsied each lesion before treatment. Sometimes I've found oncocytoma and sometimes I've found grade 2 clear cell renal cell carcinoma.

He's now nearing retirement and has been allowed to continue his profession after a brief period of disability after his open surgery. Each time I see him, we discuss the fact that at some point on some day he may require removal of his kidney. However, for the past three visits, he has had only three tiny tumors within the kidney and they have remained stable. I decided that due to their small size and appearance that these are oncocytomas. He has no evidence of anything large and growing in his kidney at this point. The largest of the original tumors was 3 cm. The remaining tumors were all very small, between ½ cm and 2½ cm.

He has nothing in his kidney now larger than about 1.8 cm. We always discuss the fact that, from the literature and from what we know about von Hippel Lindau syndrome which is a genetic syndrome which causes clear cell renal cell carcinoma, the critical size at which we start to be concerned about renal cell carcinoma becoming a serious possibility and being able to metastasize is around 3 cm. So, he is well aware that if he ever has a finding of a tumor that is approaching 3 cm., he may require additional procedures, may even require removal of his kidney. Slowly, over the past few years he has become accustomed to the information and accepting of the possibility. That doesn't prevent him from becoming nervous but he's more accepting of the potential of dialysis at some time.

The last two patients are both women. Kidney cancer is more common in men than women but, for some reason, the incidence in women is steadily increasing. The first of these two patients was 48 years old but looked more like she was 38 years old. She was a busy, vital working mother who came to see me after being diagnosed elsewhere with a very large right renal mass. Her tumor was large enough that she was diagnosed because of pain which is very unusual. She didn't have any blood in the urine. She didn't have any other side effects from her tumor, just pain in her back and pain in her right side.

We got a complete set of images on her and did find evidence of pulmonary nodules in addition to the large mass in the abdomen. I had the same discussion with her that I do with all kidney cancer patients about metastatic kidney cancer. She understood that surgery alone would not be curative and that she would need to have additional treatment afterwards if we were to have any hope of having a significant impact on her disease but that surgery was likely beneficial in the equation.

This patient is perhaps one of the most stoic people I remember ever treating. She wanted to do everything possible. Her young adult children accompanied her and agreed that they also wanted to do everything possible. We reviewed the films which showed relatively minimal pulmonary nodules. However, the right renal mass was extremely large. It looked as if it was pushing up on the liver. Kidney tumors rarely invade the liver so this is not usually a concern. There was some adenopathy or enlarged lymph nodes in the retroperitoneum in the expected location of nodal spread of a right kidney cancer but, based on both a CT scan and a MRI, this appeared to be non-problematic and easily resected. The right renal mass appeared to be abutting the duodenum and the colon but not invading either one. We had a long discussion about the potential surgery.

She went to surgery one week later. At that time, her most recent imaging was nine days old. She had a transabdominal, sub costal approach as I've previously described. Immediately upon entering the abdomen, I saw that I was not going to be able to help this woman because she had cancer studding the entire inside of her belly. This condition is called carcinomatosis. In this woman's case, there was an obvious tumor growing along the underside of the abdominal wall, completely coating it. There were fingerlike projections of tumor coming off of every single piece of her intestines. The tumor had grown into the liver and had encased the duodenum, the first portion of the small intestine. It was encroaching on but not yet invading the colon. The tumor itself was extremely fixed. We started biopsying the tumors. Everything we biopsied was indeed cancer. It was all grade 4 sarcomata renal cell carcinoma which is an extremely aggressive form of renal cell carcinoma.

I moved things around as best I could but it was immediately apparent that there was no way to feasibly remove the large tumor without taking a large portion of liver, probably removing a large portion of the duodenum, and possibly resecting a large segment of the vena cava. Several of my colleagues, one from colorectal surgery, one from general surgery, and one from vascular surgery, all agreed that the surgery would not only be extremely risky but also unlikely to be of much benefit to the patient. At this point, I asked the nurses to bring her family to the surgery operating room waiting room. I scrubbed out of surgery to discuss the situation with them. When I explained that I was unable to remove the tumor, the family became distraught. I explained that surgery would likely be more harmful than helpful in this case. The family agreed. I returned to surgery and we closed her abdomen and sent her to the hospital floor for recovery. I waited until she was fully awake and spoke with the patient.

Upon hearing the news that her tumor was still in, she simply looked away and didn't say anything more. She never really did talk to me for the remainder of her hospitalization which, thankfully for her, was brief. I did keep trying to engage her but she would not discuss anything. I explained to her why the tumor was not removed and what she needed to do to get over the immediate surgery. I had colleagues from medical oncology visit with her several times during her hospitalization. She left the hospital and was scheduled to meet with a medical oncologist closer to home. However, she had a rapid series of problems and, unfortunately, died within about five weeks of her discharge.

In contrast is the next patient, another young woman, 54 years old, with several medical problems including diabetes, hypertension, renal insufficiency, and a recently discontinued long-term history of smoking. She was admitted to a hospital after what appeared to be a massive pulmonary embolism. She was transferred to the urology service when the CT scan to look for clots in the lungs showed that she had a large renal mass with a tumor thrombus that extended into the renal vein and up the vena cava to approximately the level of the diaphragm. The tumor thrombus obviously had broken loose at this point. Previously, it must have been up significantly higher. There just appeared to be a sheared surface at approximately the level of the diaphragm and massive amounts of the tumor which had broken off were filling up the arteries of both lungs. She needed to have surgery immediately.

I went to meet with the family and to discuss the case with one of our cardiac surgeons. I met with the family for approximately two hours, discussing the fact that without surgery she would surely pass away within a very short time frame but that I was not at all sure that the surgery would be curative. Rather, the surgery itself would cause her substantial risk. I vividly remember explaining all of this to the patient herself who asked some very pertinent questions. However, at the time she was requiring a large amount of oxygen support, had quite labored breathing, and was in a significant amount of pain. She and her family members did indicate to me, however, that they did want to proceed with surgery and take any chance that we could improve her length of life. I had a lengthy discussion with a cardiac surgeon who specializes in removing clots from within pulmonary arteries.

Just so you can visualize it, this tumor had grown up the vena cava, broken off, traveled up to and through the right side of the heart and was pumped from the right side of the heart through the blood vessels into her lungs, filling up a large portion of the pulmonary arteries. This is problematic, of course, because it puts a significant strain on the heart but, more importantly, it means a large part of the lungs is not usable for exchange of gases because they're not getting blood flow. This causes significant problems with breathing. The cardiac surgeon thought he could remove a large portion of the pulmonary emboli. We both agreed however that this would be a significantly risky procedure and he expressed to the family his concerns that the surgery itself could prove lethal. Both the patient and the family were resolute in their desire to proceed with the surgery.

The next day the patient was brought to the operating room. This is a complicated surgery so she had an EEG monitor placed on her head to monitor her brain waves and a transesophageal echocardiogram, an ultrasound probe which is passed down through the esophagus, to monitor both her heart and the vena cava tumor thrombus during the surgery. Both the cardiac surgery team and my surgery team operated simultaneously. We exposed the right kidney and completely exposed the vena cava through a chevron transabdominal approach. I isolated the left renal artery. I isolated the vena cava below the tumor thrombus which was a very large, fat tumor thrombus within the vena cava. The cardiac surgeon placed the patient on a cardiac bypass machine. The patient was cooled down to 18 degrees centigrade. At multiple points during the cardiac portion of the operation, the patient's blood flow from the cardiac bypass machine was slowed to an extremely low rate so that the cardiac surgeon could open the pulmonary arteries and pull out from within them, the tumor. On two occasions, for a grand total of eighteen minutes, one 10 minute and one 8 minute time period, the patient was in a cooled state subjected to complete arrest of flow. That is, her blood was thinned and the heart bypass machine was simply stopped. During the first ten minute time period of complete circulatory arrest, I removed tumor from the vena cava while the cardiac surgeon was removing tumor from the pulmonary arteries. I was able to remove the tumor from within the vena cava completely, inspect, and close the vena cava. He finished that portion of his pulmonary embolectomy. Flow was restarted and, with flow, the remainder of her tumor mass in the belly was removed. I completed the lymphadenectomy and was then able to scrub out of the room while the cardiac surgery team continued with the pulmonary embolectomies.

At the conclusion of their procedure, she was successfully brought off the heart bypass machine, her brain waves returned to normal, and she woke up completely normally. She was then transferred to the cardiac intensive care unit. She was quite sedated until the second day after surgery. At that point she was breathing normally and was up and walking. She and I sat down and had a talk. After about ten minutes of discussing her surgery and our expectations for her, she looked at me strangely and said she had no clue who I was and didn't recall ever meeting me or discussing anything prior to her surgery. After I got over my surprise, we had a good laugh about that and we proceeded to review and discuss everything.

She did extremely well after that and left the hospital after five days. Following her discharge, she has been back to see me three times at two month intervals. She has completely normal ability for exercise for someone in her age range. She has developed no obvious metastases. Her lungs are dramatically improved and there is no more evidence of pulmonary emboli. However, she is well aware of the fact that it is extremely unlikely that we were able to remove all of her pulmonary emboli and that the radiographic images probably are inaccurate in that she probably does have residual tumor that we will see develop in her lungs. For now, she is quite grateful that she has additional time with her family and has been able to return to her normal activities, knowing that her initial visit to the hospital could have ended in death within a few days or weeks.

She has educated herself on renal cell carcinoma and has already decided that if she does have obvious evidence of development of metastatic disease she will proceed with immunotherapy. She also wants to be considered for clinical trials if she does prove to have metastatic disease. She is fully aware of the statistics for metastatic renal cell carcinoma but has explained to me that she fully intends to visit me for the next twenty to thirty years and that she is going to beat the odds. And, if anybody can do it, I can suspect that she can.

I hope that you have garnered from this chapter not only an understanding of the urologic oncologist's role in renal cell carcinoma but also an appreciation of the courage and strength of the patients with whom I am privileged to work.

NOTES:

NOTES:

CHAPTER 2

The Internist's Tumor
by Cynthia Chauhan

"The Internist's Tumor" is what Dr. A., the urologist, called the renal cell carcinoma that, undetected, has quietly grown in my body until found accidentally, or incidentally as physicians like to say.

I had had major abdominal surgery on June 4. On the morning of June 11, I awoke to unrelenting nausea and stomach pain. When the pain had not abated by early evening, Dr. O., the endocrinologist, sent me to the emergency room. After eight hours in the emergency room and a number of investigative and palliative procedures and observations, the emergency room resident decided to do an ultrasound scan. I overheard him tell another physician he didn't know what to do—If he hadn't been bawled out the night before for a precipitous discharge, he'd let me go home. But, he wanted to err on the side of caution to protect himself. Consequently, he ordered an ultrasound that incidentally revealed a sizeable mass on my right kidney. In reporting the growth to me, he was very careful to call it a mass. I felt a cold chill flow through me and asked, "Do I have cancer?" He responded that he really couldn't say.

Tenacious, I pushed, "Can't say or won't?"

"I really can't," he countered. "Further tests are indicated. Call your physician in the morning. He'll have our findings and will set up the necessary tests."

My first response was to laugh—was this the emergency room equivalent of "Take two aspirins and call me in the morning?" My laughter died as I became saturated with dread and fear. I knew it was cancer. I looked across the room at my son and breathed in his presence deeply. The thought of leaving him forever overwhelmed me and I sank back into myself feeling smaller and less significant than I ever had, knowing that I could die and the world would move on essentially unchanged. I was terrorized by knowing that my body could so easily and effortlessly grow my death without even alerting me to what was happening.

The simple statement "she found out she has cancer" does not begin to reveal the intense, complex emotions, thoughts, and physical reactions that rushed through me as I sat with my new knowledge. I tried to talk myself out of the certainty that this was cancer. After all, I hadn't even known the mass was there, how could I know it was cancer? I just knew, and I knew that I had to keep it contained. I started right then thinking of the mass as coated in an impenetrable shell that would protect me from it until it could be treated.

The other thought I had at the time was ironic relief for this serious, tired, young physician whom I overheard say to another physician just as he was coming into my room to give me the news about the tumor, "Whatever happened to simple cases like cellulitis?" No precipitous discharge this time. His fear-based thoroughness had yielded an important incidental finding. Isn't that humbling? A life-changing event happens to me and its label is incidental finding, sort of like stumbling on a pebble. It's just that this pebble would reform my relationship to my world and my place in it.

On Friday, Dr. O., my endocrinologist, saw me and ordered the diagnostic CT scan. He too was careful not to name the mass malignant but equally careful not to name it benign. He pointed out that we hide a lot of things within ourselves that do not readily announce themselves. I know he was speaking concretely but I thought about what an apt description that was of what we do intellectually and spiritually too.

Dr. O observed that the mass was large but well-circumscribed, a good sign. He saw no way to avoid surgery because of the size of the mass whether it was benign or malignant. We talked about the importance of my participation in and ownership of the decision-making process, making sure I own the final decisions and do so knowledgeably. As always, Dr. O not only discussed the medical possibilities but also focused on how I was feeling, how I was reacting to what I was learning about my body. This kind man sat patiently with me as I tried to absorb and understand what was happening within me. I was simply reeling from having spent three months preparing for and undergoing the extensive abdominal procedures that I had seen and experienced as such a trial. Now, just when I was incorporating that into my life, into my sense of my place in life, this news came hurtling in. I had just enough information to be frightened, not yet enough information to make concrete plans beyond the plans to garner more information through the CT scan. Dr. O promised me more conclusive answers after the scan but those answers would come from the surgeon and the planning would be done with him.

This conversation was on Friday. I would spend the weekend alone with my new awareness. My usual habit, when I confront something new is to learn as much about it as quickly as I can. This time, I decided to proceed differently. I decided to spend the weekend in meditation and willing my body to keep this intruder enclosed, shut off from the rest of me. I owned no part of this found thing and just wanted to distance myself from it as much as possible until I could be rid of it. I thought of all the wise things people think and say when they are faced with their own mortality. I had no wise or clever thoughts. I just knew I wanted to live, that it wasn't dying itself I minded, it was not being here, not seeing the sun rise, not watching the leaves turn, not looking at my son and feeling the surge of deep love rise up through me. I may not always live passionately but I knew I passionately wanted to live.

I had the CT scan early the morning of June 16. The attending staff were gentle, kind, supportive. But nothing could take away the loneliness and overwhelming ignorance I felt, lying perfectly still while the iodine warmed my insides against the chill of premonition that held me spellbound as the machine moved me back and forth through its portal and the computer-generated voice repeatedly instructed me to hold my breath and to breathe.

I met Dr. A, the urologist who would be my surgeon, at 4 p.m. that same day. A tall man with warm presence and gentle eyes, he brought quiet confidence into the room with him. He understood that I was desperate for answers, for information, and could not sit through social niceties when my future was in question. He got right down to business by showing me the CT scan and what we were dealing with. I was struck by his reference to what we were dealing with because I was feeling as though the tumor was dealing with me, that I was at the unwitting mercy of this silent killer. In that simple reference, he invited me to reframe my experience, to assert my authority. Dr. A affirmed my shock at the discovery and that the tumor was potentially life-threatening. He didn't know how long the tumor had been there or how fast it was growing. He was able to say it was a solid mass with about a 90% probability of being malignant and a 10% possibility of being benign. Never had the chasm between probability and possibility loomed so huge. To cope, I broke it down into good news and bad news. Good news: It's found, it's still apparently encapsulated, it can be handled and, hopefully, cured surgically. Bad news: I lose a kidney, probably to cancer. More good news: The other kidney's fine. Dr. A said the only way to find out if it was cancer would be to remove the right kidney—there was no way around that. He saw no evidence of spread to my lymph nodes, liver, or lungs but real knowledge of metastasis could only come with exploration during surgery. However, the apparent containment was important and fortunate. Listening to my body and having the ultrasound done was the best thing I could have done.

Throughout our conversation, I wept uncontrollably. In all of my life, at all the times I abstractly considered my own mortality, cancer was never part of any of the scenarios I created around my death. It just was not part of how I defined or understood myself at any level. Yet, here I was, cancerous. It felt unreal. Consequently, at that time I perceived the tumor as an outside, invading force. Only later would I comprehend that the tumor was a profusion of my own renal cells gone crazy—growing out of control, losing their sense of place in the community of my body and greedily assuming primacy that threatened not only my balance but also my life.

How carefully everyone I dealt with now chose their words and used cautious modifiers. These medical professionals were not cavalier saviors but cautious interveners with thorough knowledge of what threatened my life. Dr. A. was patient and gentle but sure of the path I needed to take. He explained the CT scan, showing me in close detail the enmeshment of the tumor with the kidney. He suggested surgery the next day but said he wouldn't argue with me if I needed to wait a few days to get things in order. That chilling caveat, to get things in order, underscored that my survival was at stake. I was terrified, caught in feeling betrayed by my body harboring this killer within me, not just harboring it but nurturing it.

Throughout our discussions, Dr. A was focused, factual, and sensitive to my emotional pain. He talked in detail about the surgery, explaining he'd go in through my side, remove one rib, free my kidney from its moorings and remove the entire kidney as well as part of the ureter after he had taken steps to protect me from drop metastasis which can happen during surgery. He was honest about the deep physical pain that would result from the surgery. He said an epidural would be used for pain control as well as a morphine pump. He outlined the risks of bleeding and infection. When he said he couldn't safely do the surgery with my hemoglobin as low as it was after the other surgery and he couldn't be party to delaying the surgery more than a week because of the tumor's size (the potential for metastasis was too great), we moved into new, fearful territory for me. The only alternative he saw was preoperative transfusion because I would lose at least a unit of blood during surgery. I got stuck on fear of HIV. He helped me to clarify the imminent, real danger of the tumor versus the possible, future danger of HIV infection. We talked about the relative safety of the blood supply versus the certain danger of the tumor. He said, "The best kind of tumor like this is one that's out of your body. There can be no peaceful maintenance."

I stayed with the questions about cancer, metastasis, life expectancy. He said many of my questions could only be answered once the tumor was removed and he looked at the final pathology. Then we could talk about prognosis depending on the stage and aggressiveness of the tumor. That would give more reliable information about likelihood of recurrence and spread. How easily we had moved into looking at me with a whole new language. A language which, only days before, had been alien to me now defined me.

As we had been talking, fear of radiation and chemotherapy had been wafting through my mind, tightening my stomach, loosening my bowels. Then, as part of the exploration of possibilities, he said that neither chemotherapy nor radiation was effective against kidney cancer. My only intervention hope was surgery. Suddenly, the chemotherapy and radiation I had dreaded flew from me like retreating guardian angels. I felt deserted, so alone, so bereft of choice. My only chance of cure was removal.

I asked him to talk with me about how much time I could take to adjust to the knowledge of what was happening in my body, to come to terms with my overwhelming mortality, how much time I could spend taking care of myself emotionally and healing physically from the prior surgery before the nephrectomy. I was stunned by my lack of choices as he reiterated that if I wanted to live, it really wasn't a matter of if I had the surgery but when. From his perspective, the sooner the better. He offered to do the surgery the next morning at 8 a.m. and said that that was his preference and recommendation. But, he understood I might need some processing time as long as I could agree to waiting no longer than a week.

My tears had been flowing freely throughout our interview but when he asked me to choose a day for surgery I shrank away within myself, feeling completely incapacitated to make any decision. He gently comforted me, offering understanding of my pain, affirming my emotional crying with the observation that my response to this news was not only normal but useful. It meant I was working on clearing my slate, accepting my newly realized reality.

Dr. A asked if I wanted to meet again on Thursday. When I could only barely whisper that I didn't know what I wanted, he offered to decide for me that we would meet in two days. In the meantime, he suggested that I work on integrating all I'd learned today. He again affirmed the healthiness of experiencing my feelings and offered to go ahead and schedule the surgery for the following Tuesday. I could always cancel it. He said these things gently and supportively, not autocratically.

We talked more about the seriousness of the tumor and the surgery, the abruptness of the situation, and my feelings of vulnerability. He agreed that I was in a very vulnerable position but he reiterated that he was confident that I'd get through the surgery, reminding me of how well I was doing after the other major surgery. He reminded me the tumor was encapsulated and that gave us a good shot at a cure. He affirmed a week would be soon enough but longer would be problematic and again encouraged me to direct my energy to working through my feelings. He'd take care of the mechanics of getting me through each step of dealing with the tumor.

I was left after that interview with confronting my finitude, accepting my fear, planning and initiating my survival. Dr. A's confidence in his ability to intervene in my best interest, his willingness to accept respectful responsibility for procedural decisions freed me to hope, to begin to feel some returning capacity to steer my own course, to retrieve ownership of my life from the tumor—in his words, to deal with it. The feelings of spinning out of control, of being at the mercy of unspeakable forces began to subside in his calm, supportive, knowledgeable presence. His kindness supplanted my hopelessness, his professionalism kindled my self-caretaking. I looked deeply at him, wanting to memorize the face and hands of this man who affirmed my dread-filled fear and, at the same time, held out bright hope. I wanted to map the hands that would enter my body searching out and removing this cancer. I took a deep breath, blew my nose, wiped my eyes. I determined to learn more about what was going on inside of me, to plan my immediate future, realizing the immediate future might be my only future.

I had just climbed to the summit of what I thought was the highest mountain only to discover it was merely a foothill of a truly high mountain. Now I had to begin the difficult course of reclaiming ownership of myself from the usurpative tumor. I was sad. I was angry. I was tired. But, clearly, the tumor would not wait.

I spent the next two days alternating between sitting and crying from a deep place within me, crying that went far beyond sadness to existential longing, and working to learn everything I could about renal cell carcinoma and the surgery I was facing. I thought about what to do with the basic knowledge that I was probably dealing with cancer and I knew I wanted the love and support of my family and friends. I called people I love, told them what I was facing, and asked for their prayers and support. They were uniformly wonderful and loving in their responses. I envisioned them helping me to keep the capsule tightly sealed, a neat package for Dr. A to remove quickly and easily.

I wrote a guided imagery for myself and listened to it for several hours each day, falling asleep as it played repeatedly through the night. I drew pastels of my body and the tumor. I read journals, pamphlets, books, articles. Knowledge did give me power. I learned what an unpredictable kind of cancer renal cell is. It's different from other cancers in that it, along with melanoma, is responsible for most spontaneous remissions. But, it is also notoriously unresponsive to interventions and can hide, undetected, for years until it has metastasized into favorite areas including bone, lungs, and brain. The usual discovery of the tumor is either accidental while looking for something else—hence the name, "the internist's tumor"—or after metastasis, when urine turns red with blood.

I directed my energy to strengthening my body through healthy eating and very mild exercise, walking, lifting soup cans for weights. I was still weak from the prior surgery but determined to go into this one as strong as possible and to become a competent, knowledgeable survivor. I was exquisitely aware of the beauty and gift of each moment of my life, of the marriage of simplicity and complexity in the marvelous world, of how very much I love being alive and want to stay alive for a long time.

On Thursday, Dr. A and I met again. We talked about what I'd been learning in the eternity since Tuesday. Dr. A said, "Information can only be helpful in adjusting to this shocking news. I have an idea of what you are going through trying to absorb all the news and the process you are involved in." It touched me that he said he had "an idea". That was so respectful of the uniqueness of my experience. To me, it was acknowledgement that no one else could know my feelings and experience exactly as well as confirmation of his willingness to stay open to my needs and perceptions. He said he hoped that I was planning to live a long life because he was planning to help me to do that. Those simple words affirmed my potential to move through this crisis into a healthier future. It is those small observations that are so encouraging when life is darkened by present crisis. No promises, just hope and companionship.

Trying to avert any unnecessary losses, I asked if he had to take my rib. He said it was safer to go in that way because of the size of the mass and the need to thoroughly explore the region. We talked about staging the tumor (determining how advanced it was and the extent of any metastasis) and whether or not he would remove lymph nodes and my adrenal gland. He said staging would be done post-removal and that he'd have to decide once he was inside whether or not to remove the adrenal gland and any lymph nodes. His best guess now was that the adrenal gland and the lymph nodes were not yet involved and wouldn't have to be removed. But, he cautioned me, that was an educated guess, not a factual statement. We talked about the necessity of blood transfusion and the accompanying risk of HIV infection. He laughed when I told him I'd been eating liver religiously and then pointed out there's quite a long wait for eating liver to affect blood levels. It felt good that we could laugh together and still stay focused on the work at hand. He reassured me again about the relative safety of the blood supply. We agreed that life is about risks and the risk of the tumor far outweighed the risk of the transfusion. He could see no way around transfusion so I'd check into the hospital Monday, be transfused through the night, and surgery would be Tuesday.

Dr. A closed the interview by saying, "We're going to get you through this." The "we're" was an irresistible invitation to join with him in acting in my own best interest. There was a sureness in his voice when he said that that I grabbed onto and wrapped around my heart to sustain me. He was certain of his skill. I was afraid but learning to mediate my fear with knowledge and trust. Looking back, I know that more than his words, his demeanor of confidence, skill, and empathy had a strong, calming effect on me. His confidence did not edge over into arrogance. He never suggested that I just entrust myself to him. He did not supplant my autonomy with his authority. Rather, he supported my search for knowledge, spoke of the two of us working together to overcome this problem, gave me his warm, compassionate presence to draw upon, to use to strengthen myself. Through his confidence in his skill and understanding of my fear and bewilderment, he lent me strength until I could rebuild my own resources.

Surgery was scheduled for the following Tuesday. That gave me four more days to build my physical strength and my emotional and mental readiness. I used that time wisely, continuing to meditate, draw, write, and listen to my guided imageries. I continued working to build my physical strength through walking and lifting soup cans. I talked with people who loved me and drew their love and strength into myself. Through it all, I cried. Gradually my crying changed from overflowing tears of anguish to cleansing tears of transcendence. They welled up from and flowed out of the depth of my being.

My son, Jai, was with me throughout this ordeal, as he had been through the earlier surgery. My husband, Om, and I have a small business which the two of us run. It wasn't feasible for both of us to be gone the four weeks we thought I would be away. We also didn't consider it feasible to have the procedure done locally. The three of us talked and decided that Jai would go with me to take care of me through the surgery and recovery period. We anticipated a routine major surgery and recovery period for which I was well-prepared physically and emotionally.

Instead, Jai was there when the emergency room resident told me of the incidental finding. Jai patiently sat by my side as I worked to own the changes I was going through. Jai took me to the hospital and held me up when my knees buckled in fear.

On the second anniversary of the nephrectomy, I asked Jai to talk with me about what it had been like for him to caretake me through those first weeks of my cancer journey. He said it was a privilege, albeit a painful, ambivalent one. He said he would not have been anywhere else even though there were times he had to get away to restore himself. He reminded me that he was there for me but there was no one there for him. He talked about the difficulty of taking care of someone whom you love when you can't offer even palliation, only witness.

I asked him about his fear about me dying. He said he didn't fear my dying. He knew my death could be imminent but he knew that even if I died he would survive and do well. He reminded me that when I came out of the recovery room after the first surgery I had lost so much blood that I was deathly white and difficult to rouse to consciousness. He said that sitting by my bedside through that, watching nurses try unsuccessfully to get me to respond, had devastatingly confronted him with my mortality. It was then that he knew that when I died he would always carry me in his heart and head. He would miss my physical presence but my spiritual presence would endure.

Jai wondered if the cancer experience would have been harder on him if he hadn't already been caring for me. He reminded me that I was terribly weakened and in persistent pain already. He reminded me of how intense and severely limiting the pain from the first surgery was. I realized I had forgotten that, swept away as I was by the far greater emotional pain of the cancer and physical pain of the nephrectomy. It seems that I can hold onto only so much awareness of pain and survive.

Jai said, "I probably ran on automatic pilot much of the time because the pain for me was overwhelming. You are my mom and I love you. To be constantly present at your suffering did make me want to run away; to pretend, even for a few moments, that none of this was real. That's when I'd go out for coffee. Then, as soon as I left, I wanted to run back to your side."

Jai got some small relief when Om, my mother, and my Uncle Willie came to be with me the day before the nephrectomy and stayed until the day after. Like Jai, they were truly strengthening. They loved and cuddled me, distracting me with delightful stories of our lives together, encouraging me with stories of past tests overcome. They were patient with me when I turned away from their love and withdrew into myself searching for meaning and understanding. Most importantly, they were there, willing me to survive.

Although I had home-nursing care to help me with physical care, Jai gave me the loving care that comes from the presence of a beloved person witnessing inescapable experience. His presence increased my fortitude, my determination to reclaim my life.

By Monday when I checked into the hospital I was feeling peaceful and ready for surgery. I just wanted to be rid of the mass that I envisioned as a black spot and to continue working on my health. For eleven days, from that moment in the emergency room when the young physician said there was a mass, I had committed myself to working to compress that hard black spot, to keeping it encapsulated until it could be removed. I saw it as a black shell encapsulating a deadly white embryonic parasite. I visualized the black shell as seamless and strong. I had come to understand I must sacrifice my right kidney to be rid of this death seed. My healthy left kidney would easily assume all renal function for me. I felt grateful to my right kidney for the good work it had done for fifty-six years. I would have liked to take my kidney home and bury it but Dr. A had explained to me that the hospital would not release it to me because staff needed it for on-going access. So, I decided to say goodbye to this important part of me in the operating room and to frame it as a sacrificial leave-taking for the greater good of my whole body. It was clear to me that removal of my kidney was essential to my continued survival.

As I walked into the hospital, a wave of sheer terror flooded me, my knees buckled, I saw everything around me in startling detail. I was acutely aware of being awash in a sea of non-choices masquerading as hard choices. I had spent the whole day drinking in everything my eyes saw, imprinting the beauty of being alive in every cell of my being.

Deep sadness at my loss of innocence washed over me too. Cancer deprived me of a primal innocence, a trust in my knowledge of my own body that now lost could never be retrieved. I pay attention to my body, listen closely to its messages but I know concretely that sometimes important things, life-altering things are happening inside of me and my body acquiesces silently while my mind remains ignorant. The worst seed that cancer has planted is the omnipresent certainty that no matter how conscious I am, on a cellular level my body goes its own way and carries within it the code of its own destruction. This is something everyone knows theoretically. The knowledge is different when it is concrete experience with one's own body. That's what I appreciated so much when Dr. A said, "I have an idea of what you're going through" rather than "I know." The first is an offering of presence with me, the second is arrogance.

The hospital stay is a blur of pain experienced, relieved, reexperienced. The nephrectomy was an intensely painful surgery. A major nerve had been cut, a rib removed, and my insides pushed and probed, first to make room for a clear, clean removal of the kidney and tumor, then to look for metastasis in surrounding tissue and organs. Sharp pain, burning pain, aching pain, movement pain, stationary pain cascaded through me. The epidural pain block provided salutary relief so great that I thought I had handled the surgery really well. Then I was removed from the epidural and plunged into a pit of extreme, unremitting pain that responded to IV and oral medications but never ceased. The medications fogged my mind and slowed my body but the pain swept on. I learned about levels of pain, about trading symptoms for side effects, about how pain filters and alters reality. I worked hard on accepting the pain, relaxing into it rather than fighting it. That was helpful in getting through the pain but for about four weeks pain clearly controlled my life.

During that time, actually on the Friday after surgery, I lost Dr. A for a while. He was transferred to another hospital within the system and I was bereft. I had allowed myself to lean on him, to trust him to see me through this whole process. I guess we had different definitions of what that meant. He had seen me through the surgery, visited me daily through Friday, given me the pathology report: Stage 2, no lymph node involvement, no apparent metastasis, and would see me again as an outpatient but the rest of my hospitalization would be supervised by a different surgeon. I had thought I would be seen exclusively by Dr. A until my discharge from urology service. Realistically, in retrospect, I understand the difference in our experiences of our therapeutic relationship and that Dr. A had been there for me in the important, life-saving ways. It was just that I had spent the month of June being stripped of important aspects of myself and was unusually vulnerable to any loss.

It was easy to replace my experience of loss with feelings of abandonment, to short-circuit the work I had to do to come to terms with the redefinition of my body that I was experiencing. When I thought about it carefully, I was able to refocus on taking responsibility for myself and my own recovery. Dr. A had done what he had set out to do, to free my body from cancer. Now, it was up to me to free myself from it. That has taken much longer. And I'm not really free of it—I suspect I never will be. Each time I go for a check-up I move into a breathless, suspended reality when the terror sweeps through me as I sit with the knowledge that I have no idea what's going on inside of me. I am acutely aware of my ignorance. I only hope. Now, I know the cancer as part of who I am--part of my uniqueness. It has reified my mortality. The gift that has flown from this dreadful experience is constant awareness of the precious fragility, the fragile preciousness of my life and of my responsibility to live my life as a sacred experience. I am but a moment on the breath of the divine. It is up to me to cherish my moment. I watch the autumn leaves skirmish on the lawn and dance through the neighborhood, seemingly alive and I think about this dance of life in which I am blown about by the winds of fate. My choices are not so much what happens to me as how I choose to react to the forces of life. What holds my dignity? What shapes my character?

On July 14, I saw Dr. A again. I was happy to be back in his presence. I had let go of the feelings of abandonment as I regained my strength. My head had always understood, my emotions had simply reacted. Part of wholeness for me is accepting all of the diversity of response within myself and processing it into who I am. At this visit I was concerned about the ongoing intense pain. It was unrelenting, constant, and unaffected by doses of pain medicine that I was willing to take. The pain at the front of the fourteen inch incision was sharp and stabbing. Along the incision line and radiating out it was burning. At the back it was constant burning and aching. I was worn down by its omnipresence. Dr. A affirmed the aftermath of this surgery was typically very pain filled for about eight weeks because of the size and depth of the incision as well as the rib removal and probing of the surrounding area. He said the nerves along the right side were irritated by the surgery because they'd been pushed around quite a bit and some had had to be cut. There are only so many ways my nerve fibers can signal pain—sharp, burning, dull. Different pain receptors tell the brain to feel things in different ways. Cutting through hits all of the receptors, firing them all. It takes time for them to settle down but finally they stop. It's a matter of waiting through it.

We talked about the conflict between enduring pain and tolerating the side effects of the pain medications. The pain medications dulled my mind and slowed my gastro-intestinal tract miserably. I hated the dullness. I have always experienced my mind as my most precious part of self and just plain enjoyed thinking. The medicines robbed me of that. Also, the dullness was counter to my new appreciation of the precious beauty of each moment. There was no more ordinary in my life. Common encounters shone with the fiery beauty of rare jewels.

Dr. A worked with me to help me to reframe the inescapable pain. First, I acknowledged that while it was inescapable, it was not unendurable. I willingly acknowledged I was choosing less relief to keep my mind alert and to continue working on strengthening my body. Second, although I was experiencing the pain as overwhelming, it was, in fact, running a normal course, just a very trying course. My work now was to hold onto the source of the pain, freedom from cancer, as a way of tolerating the pain. We talked about distracting myself and gradually increasing my physical activity.

Through all of this conversation, Dr. A was supportive and comforting. His voice was gentle and comforting, his demeanor concerned and attentive. He reminded me that, while we were working together as a team, my experience was uniquely mine. He could not free me from it but he was there to help me to face it and to interpret the physical experience for me. The comforting presence of another human being is a strong palliation for pain. It doesn't decrease the physical experience but it tempers the emotional response and bolsters tolerance.

I did not see Dr. A again until the following April. In the meantime, my recovery and care was supervised by an internist, Dr. M. When I did see Dr. A again, we spent most of that visit talking about renal cell carcinoma and the importance of lifelong vigilance even when surgical removal has been apparently successful. By the time we met again, my Aunt Lillian had been diagnosed with metastasized renal cell carcinoma and had died a long, painful death as the metastasis was to her brain and spinal cord. Fifteen years earlier, my Aunt Hilda had had a small renal cell carcinoma and one of her kidneys removed. That made three women in my family with this malignancy which strikes rarely and then usually older male smokers.

Dr. A neither soft-pedaled the truth nor used it as a club. He spoke simply and straightforwardly, neither dodging difficult questions nor using them as springboards for pontification. He was patient. He understood that simple information can be loaded with meanings that make it difficult to take in all at once. In response to my questions, Dr. A talked about what I need to stay alert to: poor appetite, unexplained weight loss, or if something, anything, just doesn't feel right. He told me that this tumor had been a moderately aggressive cancer. That meant that if there were recurrences we would have time to intervene. He emphasized the importance of a healthy diet with less than sixty grams per day of protein to protect my remaining kidney. He said kidney cancer, even when we think we've achieved surgical cure, is a cancer that has to be monitored for the rest of my life. It's been known to recur as much as twenty-five years later and there are no good therapies except removal. Close monitoring allows early detection and removal. He reinforced the need for close monitoring as he talked about what a tough, nasty cancer renal cell is when it spreads. As my Aunt Lillian had experienced, even pain relief is difficult.

I left that interview with some despair. Never again could I just assume I was healthy. Always lurking in my depths might be a stray renal cell fallaciously, fatally encoded.

I saw Dr. A one more time at the end of June, my one-year survival anniversary. We were both upbeat about my prospects. He was interested in how I was putting my life back together and supportive of my ability to keep myself focused on important health issues. If anything, the cancer affirmed a conscious, thoughtful lifestyle in which I practiced healthy eating and rebuilt my ability to exercise. I regained my movement and exercise abilities slowly but I did regain them. I learned about foods that are protective against cancer and made sure to include generous servings in my daily meals

Following that interview, Dr. A. transferred me back to internal medicine for long term follow-up. The gift I received from Dr. A was no less than my life. The lesson I learned from him is the value of calm competence in meeting the trials of life. He validated my right to my own feelings, my responsibility to myself to define the role of cancer in my life, my ability to survive.

For three years, I did very well. My internist researched the appropriate follow-up protocol for kidney cancer and followed it meticulously. But, three years out from my kidney cancer, I was diagnosed with breast cancer. As part of that routine follow up, enlarged para aortic lymph nodes and nodules on one of my lungs were found. I went into a tailspin. I began, once again, to do my own research on kidney cancer and to understand that, no matter how good my internist is, and he is very, very good, I should be followed by someone specializing in renal cell carcinoma. My internist still manages and supervises my care, coordinating the findings of the specialists I see for multiple health problems, focusing his own expertise and wisdom on my health issues. A renal cell carcinoma specialist has been added to my health care team.

The person I found is a urologic oncologist. He thoroughly reviewed my CT scans and my history as well as the pathology of my tumor. Observing the nodes and nodules and looking back at all of my CT scans, he determined that they are stable and that resection of the nodes would be riskier than watching them. The nodules are too small for removal and stable. He believes they are unlikely to be rcc metastasis but continues observation. The vital thing that I learned from this crisis is that not only is it important to have regular follow-up for the rest of my life—Dr. A. had engrained that in me—but also that the follow up should be by a physician specialized in renal cell carcinoma, either a urologic oncologist or a medical oncologist with a special interest and expertise in renal cell carcinoma.

NOTES:

CHAPTER 3
The Oncologist's Role *in the* Management *of* Renal Cell Carcinoma
by Jaime Merchan, M.D.

The medical oncologist has an important role in kidney cancer. We need not only to fight cancer but also to learn from it, to break down walls and barriers, to work together to expand our boundaries. This discussion of the role of medical oncology in kidney cancer is divided into three sections. The first section is a general review of the role of the oncologist and what you should look for in an oncologist. The second section reviews the current standard therapies, including IL2 and interferon, and discusses the continuing role of IL2 in treatment of kidney cancer as new therapies emerge. The third section focuses on novel therapies, including antiangiogenic therapies, concluding with a brief discussion of the promise of the future in which patients will receive individualized treatments based on their tumor's characteristics.

THE ONCOLOGIST *and* RENAL CELL CARCINOMA

Why should patients with renal cell cancer see an oncologist? What's important about that? What should patients expect when meeting with a medical oncologist? What should they ask? Is it better to wait until after the nephrectomy to talk to an oncologist or should an oncologist become involved as soon as kidney cancer is suspected?

Ideally, the first visit should be with both the medical oncologist and the urologist, in a multidisciplinary approach where the urologist talks about the surgical part and the medical oncologist begins to make plans with the patient about what will happen after surgery. In this approach, the patient leaves the office with the sense of a plan, knowing exactly what to do and what the options are, including and after surgery.

It is vital that the oncologist be experienced in kidney cancer so that you are getting the most up-to-date information on kidney cancer, not only in terms of new discoveries regarding behaviors of the tumors but more importantly in terms of the potential and most up-to-date treatment options. It is very important that you ask the oncologist about his level of experience with kidney cancer. Choosing a medical oncologist experienced in dealing with kidney cancer improves the probability that you will get accurate information and state of the art care. While there will be questions that any oncologist may not be able to answer just because there is no answer, you will get better information from an oncologist who works with kidney cancer on a regular basis. Take the time to find an oncologist who is experienced in treating kidney cancer because so much is changing so quickly in the current directions of treatment. You have the right to question the expertise of your physicians.

When the patient has metastatic renal cell cancer, the discussion with the oncologist should include eventual treatment options. Certainly, there have been cases where just taking the main tumor out initiates subsidizing and regression of the metastases but that occurs in less than one percent of the patients. When a patient has metastases that are not causing any immediate danger, waiting and watching may be an option if the patient is ambivalent about toxic treatments. The oncologist and the patient also need to talk about the long term prognosis and recurrence risk.

One of the most difficult questions that the patient asks is, "What are the chances that the cancer will come back or that my tumors may progress and that will give me problems or kill me?" That is a very difficult question because kidney cancer is a very heterogeneous disease. While some tumors may be fast growing, there are patients in whom the tumors grow very slowly or not at all for some time. The only way to know that is with regular checkups with imaging studies.

When a patient with metastatic renal cell cancer (RCC) comes to my clinic, I discuss three potential management options, and the decision as to which one is better for the patient depends on each case. Depending on the number and size of metastases, and also depending on the patient's health and functional status, the physician will determine whether treatment is needed sooner rather than later. One option is standard therapy, which includes immune based treatments, such as IL-2 and/or interferon. The second option is enrollment into clinical trials with novel agents or novel treatment strategies. The third option is watchful waiting, where no active treatment is administered and patients are followed with imaging studies. In this case, at each visit a discussion regarding the necessity to start treatment should take place between patient and physician, based on evidence of tumor progression or on symptoms. It is very important that discussions between the patient and the oncologist include the benefits and risks of each of the treatment options. Ask about clinical trials because they are especially important in kidney cancer. Including them in the discussion is the only way the doctors will know what treatments are best for you and you can make truly informed decisions about the treatment options.

Once you have a relationship with an oncologist who is experienced in treating kidney cancer, you are ready to begin discussing your options.

STANDARD TREATMENTS *for* METASTATIC RENAL CELL CANCER

SURGERY

The role of removing the primary tumor in the kidney has been reviewed earlier in Chapter 1. In some patients who present with distant metastases (outside the kidney), removal of the metastatic sites (metastatectomy) may be recommended. This procedure is usually reserved to patients whose metastases have not significantly changed over time, and who are good surgical candidates. The reason for removing metastases in selected patients with renal cell cancer is that this procedure may be associated with long term survival. The factors that are associated with prolonged survival after surgery are not entirely known, but may include having only one site of metastases (especially lung) as opposed to more than one, a very good functional status, and a disease free interval (time without tumor recurrence) after surgery of more than one year. It is important that a patient with metastatic renal cell cancer discusses the option for surgery with his oncologist and surgeon.

RADIATION THERAPY

The role of radiation therapy in the treatment of metastatic renal cell cancer is limited. Radiation therapy is usually given for palliative purposes (to relieve symptoms) in patients with tumors metastatic to the bones or to the brain.

SYSTEMIC THERAPY

This discussion will focus mainly on systemic therapies for metastatic clear cell carcinoma, the most common type of kidney cancer. Current standard treatment for patients with metastatic disease is immune based treatments, with drugs such as interleukin-2 and interferon.

Interleukin-2 (IL-2) is currently the only FDA approved treatment for metastatic renal cell cancer. The mechanism of antitumor effects of IL-2 is not entirely understood, but it is believed to enhance the function of lymphocytes (a type of immune cells that are important in mediating antitumor effects). IL-2 can be administered either intravenously or subcutaneously. Different doses and regimens have been used. However, the regimen that has been associated with higher response rates, and even with complete responses (complete disappearance of the tumors) is intravenous high dose IL-2. The overall response rate for high dose IL-2 ranges between 15 and 20%. Approximately 8% of patients enjoy a more complete response that can be long lasting (years). High dose IL-2, however, is associated with significant toxicity (which requires patients to be closely monitored in an intensive care unit for management of side effects), which makes this therapy restricted to healthy patients with an excellent functional status and normal organ function. Current research efforts are focused on discovering tumor characteristics and factors that can predict response to IL-2. Identification of those factors will help physicians determine which patients with metastatic renal cell cancer will benefit the most from high dose IL-2.

Interferon alpha (IFNα) is another immune based treatment that has been used in the treatment of patients with metastatic RCC. It has a modest antitumor activity (response rate between 10-15%), and the responses are seldom long lasting. IFN has been used both as single agent and in combination with low dose IL-2, without showing a significant increase in antitumor effects. The side effects of IFNα are in general less severe than high dose IL-2 and may include flu-like symptoms, decreased white blood cells, depression, abnormal liver tests, altered taste and depression. It is still commonly used by oncologists because of its relative safety, ease of administration, and familiarity to the community oncologist.

NOVEL THERAPIES

CHEMOTHERAPIES

Renal cell cancer is usually resistant to chemotherapy. However, recent studies have demonstrated that the combination of the chemotherapeutic agents 5FU and gemcitabine have some activity in metastatic RCC. This chemotherapy combination has produced a 15 -17% response rate. In other (non-clear cell) types of renal cell cancer chemotherapy may be one of the first options for systemic therapy. For example, in sarcomatoid renal cell cancer, a very aggressive form of kidney cancer, the combination of adriamycin and gemcitabine may have some clinical activity.

TARGETED THERAPIES

Thanks to advances in the understanding of the molecular mechanisms of renal cell cancer, a number of agents and strategies have been developed to treat this disease in a rational manner. Renal cell cancer, especially clear cell, is characterized by being a very vascularized tumor. This is due to gene defects in the tumor that lead to production of factors that stimulate blood vessel growth in a process called tumor angiogenesis. Tumor angiogenesis is a process that is vital for tumors. If angiogenesis is blocked, tumors will not grow. One of the most important factors associated with tumor angiogenesis is vascular endothelial growth factor (VEGF). For this reason, a number of agents that inhibit this factor at different levels have been evaluated in this disease.

One of the first antiangiogenic agents to be tested in metastatic RCC is Bevacizumab (Avastin, Genentech). A study in patients with metastatic RCC who progressed on standard therapies has shown that Bevacizumab delays tumor progression compared to placebo. Current studies are testing combinations of Bevacizumab with standard therapies as well as with other targeted agents. Other agents that affect angiogenesis that are in advanced stages of development include SU11248 and Sorafenib (Bay 43-9006). Recent studies have shown that these two agents are active against clear cell RCC and they may become standard treatments for RCC in the near future.

Other targeted agents that are being actively studied in RCC include CCI-779, AG 013736, erlonitib, VEGF trap, etc. These agents are being studied either alone or in combination with standard or other targeted therapies in an attempt to enhance antitumor effects.

An important consideration regarding antiangiogenic and targeted therapies is that because of the way they work, they may not eradicate the tumors (complete responses), but may prevent further tumor growth (stable disease) or cause some disease regression (partial response). For this reason, targeted therapies may need to be administered in a continuous manner in order to control the cancer.

OTHER NOVEL THERAPIES

Other treatment strategies that are being developed include treatments aimed at enhancing the patient's immune response against the cancer, such as tumor/dendritic cell vaccines and bone marrow transplant (non-myeloablative transplant), where the transplanted immune cells may attack the cancer cells. All these treatments remain investigational.

Clinical Trials

Because the above new therapies are showing promise in metastatic RCC, and because these agents are not commercially available yet, it is very important that patients with metastatic RCC ask their medical oncologists about clinical trials. It is important that a patient with metastatic RCC considers participating in clinical trials, because they may offer clinical benefit that standard treatments may not. When considering participating in clinical trials it is important that the patient carefully reads the consent form, which is a document that gives details about the treatment, the side effects, the benefits and risks of the treatment, as well as alternative options. All this information has to be provided by the consent and by the medical oncologist or investigator responsible for the clinical trial, and is important in order to make an informed decision. It is also important to emphasize that the patient is the one who makes the decision to participate, and that if a patient refuses to participate, he/she will not lose his/her rights to receive medical care by a medical institution.

Thanks to the recent advances in the treatment of metastatic RCC, the future looks promising and brings hope for patients affected by this disease. There are many agents that may show significant clinical benefit and that may improve both the patient's quality and quantity of life. Because many new potential options may become available for the treatment of RCC, current research is focused in trying to identify factors or characteristics either in the tumor or in the patient that correlate with significant clinical benefit. In the future, treatments may be "individualized", and the choice of a specific drug or combination of drugs may depend on the molecular characteristics of the individual tumor. Each tumor and each patient is unique and may respond differently to different agents. Even though we are not at that point yet, thanks to advances in medical technology, this future is not very distant.

In summary, the medical oncologist has an important role in the management of renal cell cancer at all stages of the disease. It is important that medical oncologists work together with urologists and other members of the team caring for the patient with renal cell cancer. In the last 5 years, there has been an "explosion" of new drugs that show promising clinical activity against metastatic RCC (especially clear cell RCC) and that bring new hope for patients with advanced RCC, who until recently didn't have any. Participation in clinical trials is essential to accelerate the discovery of new treatments and further improve the quality and quantity of life of our patients.

NOTES:

NOTES:

CHAPTER 4
My Politically Incorrect Cancer
by Sally LaLone

There is a lyric from a Grateful Dead song that perfectly characterizes me:

"See that girl barefooting along, whistling and singing,
she's a carryin' on..."

Carrying on. That's a nice way to put it.

I have always been a non-conformist. I never made a conscious effort to be "different." I just am.

And, frankly, I have always been proud of it. Even when it got me into trouble. Which, to be honest, it often has. I've broken all the "rules." I was always the first one on my block to try something new... like becoming a single mother in 1978. It's so humdrum now, but not when I did it! It took courage... and lots of it! I've never followed the crowd...most of the time they followed me. And if they didn't, they surely wanted to!! Who wants to be just like everyone else? Not me! Not ever!! So what if I am a bit rebellious? It doesn't change the fact that I am a warm, loving, intelligent, compassionate, empathetic, generous, kind, caring, and considerate person. Wow, there sure were a lot of adjectives in that last sentence! Maybe I should have added another...conceited or just convinced! Obviously, there's no false modesty going on here!! Truthfully, I think that those who know me best would say (after they get done laughing) that I really do have a good heart. I am also rather shy, although no one ever believes it. But, it is the truth. I just overcompensate by being brash, outrageous and (at least in my own mind) humorous. The fact is that I really love being unique!!

Well, that may not be completely true. Not anymore. In recent months, I've found that there's one very important situation in which I'd prefer to be more like other people. I've learned it isn't always a good thing to be different. I also know that there isn't anything I can do to change it. Once again, it's not a matter of choice.

As far as I know, I am the first one in my family or in my circle of friends to be stricken with something called renal cell carcinoma. Have you ever heard of it? No? Well, neither have I. It is also known as Kidney Cancer. Have you heard about that? Nope? Geez... me either. Apparently it's not a really popular topic. I think renal cell carcinoma should be officially renamed "Politically Incorrect Cancer." No one seems to know too much about it. And it is my personal belief that nobody really seems to care. Not unless this disgusting disease directly affects them. I think it is downright criminal the way kidney cancer is so unheard of! RCC is my acronym for Really Crappy Cancer!!

As you hear more about my ride on this roller coaster from hell, I think you'll see why I feel the way I do. Why, for the first time in my life, I'd like to blend in with the rest of the crowd. This time I want to fit in! I want to belong! Right now, I would give anything to be "politically correct." If there were only some magical way for me to make this change, believe me, I wouldn't hesitate—not for one split second! If only there was a magic wand or a magic pill.

Cancer is a brutal word. There is no other way to describe it. It's just plain brutal. It sucker punches you square in the belly. It knocks the wind right out of you and just sends you sprawling!! And when you are able to get back up, you find yourself living inside of a nightmare. I don't think there's anything that could ever prepare you to hear the word "Cancer." Especially in reference to yourself.

Quite honestly, it changes the way you think. It happens instantly! At least it did for me. Since my diagnosis, I've spent quite a bit of time sitting around thinking some really bizarre things. Things like...Why me? Why couldn't I just get something that everyone else has heard of?? How about something with a 95% cure rate? How about anything that someone knows about? Better statistics and mortality rates would be a really nice thing. And how about a specialist in my own area? What a convenience that would be! Instead, I have to drive more than two hours to see a doctor who is actually an expert in this despicable disease.

At one point I actually had the absurd belief that breast cancer would be a great alternative. There are foundations (whatever they are) for breast cancer...there are literally thousands upon thousands of support groups...there're the ever-present pink ribbons, there are ads everywhere that say "buy this and a portion of the proceeds will be donated to the cause"...there's breast cancer awareness month...there's surgery... then there's reconstructive surgery. And most importantly, there is chemo and radiation that have an effect on the damn disease. Caught early enough, the survival rate is phenomenal…at least compared to what I've got. I'd trade with anyone in a heartbeat!!

Please understand that I am not trying to offend anyone. But, what I have to say is not for the faint of heart…I don't mean to be insensitive to anyone else, but I really think that I got dealt a bad hand! I realize that no form of cancer is better than any other. They're all horrible. But a lot of other people have something I don't have much of... HOPE. Medical science is on their side!! I have bravado, but not really "hope."

God knows that NO cancer treatment is a walk in the park. But, there are proven medicines and therapies that enable people to live long, happy lives afterwards! Honestly, right now I would give ANYTHING to be someone who would have to spend months suffering through surgery, chemo, and radiation and have to lose my hair as long as I knew that there was a CURE! I would proudly wear scarves or wigs if I had to!! There is certainly no shame in doing that. I really wouldn't mind looking like the female version of Telly Savalas in Kojak. If that were what it took for me to get better, I'd do it with a great big smile on my face! I'd put a lollipop in my mouth and make a major fashion statement. I'd tattoo a great big cancer ribbon on my head!! How cool would that be? And then I would wait and see if my stick straight hair would grow back into the curly locks I have always dreamed of. In time, I would heal. And I would live. Which is all that really matters.

When I was first diagnosed with renal cell carcinoma, I didn't know what to do or who to talk to. While I was waiting for the barrage of tests to be done, I made myself sick and everyone else around me crazy. I needed to talk to someone who understood what I was going through. Someone who could relate to how frightened I was. And how angry. I was scared, sad, and mad all at the same time.

A friend suggested that I call a cancer help line. What a great idea! I really needed some kind of a support group. I needed to find some people who were in the same boat! Maybe we could plug the leaks and bail water together! I didn't think I could get through it by myself. I needed guidance. I needed someone to show me the ropes. But mostly, I needed some hope!

The call I made was a huge disappointment! To my complete and utter dismay, all the support groups in my area were cancer specific. Lung Cancer…Prostate Cancer...Colon Cancer...Breast Cancer. There was a long list of support groups for all kinds of diseases, but there was nothing out there for me. I didn't fit in to any of the proper categories! I was told there wasn't any general cancer support group in the local vicinity either.

I remember thinking that there is just no support for misfits. Talk about feeling left out! To make me feel even worse, besides having no support group for me to join, there were no fund raising walks, no pink ribbons, no telethons, no celebrity auctions, and no huge charity events. There was NOTHING for kidney cancer patients. Literally nothing. Not even a bake sale. And that just plain sucks!

In my opinion, part of the reason no one has heard about RCC is because there hasn't been any big celebrity who's come forward to say that either he or she or a loved one suffers from it. Off the top of my head, I can think of several stars that have battled and survived breast cancer. I know of a former big city mayor who fought and beat prostate cancer. There is another celebrity who was able to raise public awareness about colon cancer. I really wanted to thank her when my doctor recommended a colonoscopy for me!! And quite recently, there was a famous comedian who had a kidney transplant. But that isn't the same as kidney cancer. It's not even close.

Now, don't get me wrong. I think it's a very courageous and wonderful thing that these people have come forward and talked about their personal experiences, as patients or as care-givers, in order to educate the rest of us. I am thrilled for every single one of them who has been treated and has been cured. I cry along with each one of them when their story takes a bad turn and the person they are advocating for passes away. I applaud each and every one of them for sharing a bit of themselves with the rest of us. Their stories are both riveting and heart wrenching. By putting their stories out there, they raise public awareness, and they are quite often able to raise enormous amounts of money for research. Naturally, the money goes towards research of the particular cancer that touched the life of that particular celebrity. I am sure I don't have to explain to anyone why research is so important. That's how medication is developed. That's how cures are found. That's how lives are saved.

Have you ever noticed all the information given out about what I now call the Politically Correct Cancers? There are pamphlets, newspaper and magazine articles, and reports on television. There are spokespeople, benefit concerts. You name it. Not only is there public awareness for the politically correct cancers... everywhere you look you can find some information on ways to help prevent them. Eat more fiber. Drink green tea. Stay out of the sun. We all know the benefits of things like cruciferous vegetables...and flavonoids...and antioxidants. Don't forget to do self exams. Check your testicles! Buddy up for your breast exams!

Get tested! Have a colonoscopy! And those yearly pap smears aren't fun, but they aren't painful either. So, don't miss one. Make sure to have your mammograms on time...every time. And it's just common knowledge that smoking is hazardous to your health. Don't do it! Just say no!!

Because of all the information we are bombarded with, we all know how cancer is treated and cured, right? First there's the diligent doctor who actually finds the cancer. Then there's usually a biopsy. More often than not, next comes some kind of surgical procedure to remove the cancer. Afterwards, there are chemotherapy and radiation treatments. Doesn't every cancer patient have to be treated with one or the other? Sometimes both? Isn't that just the standard regimen? As long as you catch it early enough, that's how cancer is treated and cured, right? You'll be very sick for a while, and you will probably lose your hair, but, after the treatment is over, your hair grows back. And then you recover and live happily ever after, right?

Hmm... Maybe not. Not for me, anyhow.

I'm sorry. I forgot to introduce myself. My name is Sally LaLone. I am a wife and the mother of three. I have one daughter and two sons. And I wasn't kidding when I said earlier that I do things in my own way and in my own time. I became a grandmother long before I ever became a bride! My husband, Ted and I will celebrate our fourth wedding anniversary next month. My daughter, Jessica is twenty-seven, all grown up and out on her own. My sons, Daniel and Matthew are both in their early teens. Dan will be fifteen in a couple of days and Matt will be fourteen in a few months. Both of them will be in high school this fall. My granddaughter, Rebecca, who just turned nine, was the flower girl at my wedding!! Like I said, all things in my own way and in my own time.

I've never worried about getting older. I've always been healthy, so I never thought about the possibility of becoming ill. I was also blessed by looking much younger than my years. I felt no angst about my thirtieth birthday. In fact, I remember being angry because I didn't look old enough to be served a drink when my friends took me out that night. I didn't know how to drive, so I didn't have a license, no "proof" that I was of legal age to drink. And not one bouncer in Greenwich Village believed I was over twenty one, let alone thirty! It was a both a blessing and a curse!

When I hit forty, I decided it was time to grow up. I made a conscious effort to take better care of myself. I quit smoking for a year and a half. Got my nails done every week and for a while I went to a tanning salon almost every day. Probably wasn't the smartest thing I've ever done, but for me it was a daily twenty minute therapy session. Peace and quiet and no kids. A single mom's dream! I began to think of myself as a beautiful, blonde, bronzed goddess. Not too much conceit there, huh? Well, it kept me from fearing middle age. I looked about ten years younger than my chronological age! I had no trouble forgetting that I was closer to fifty than I was to twenty-five. And, over the next few years, my entire way of thinking had changed. I finally became a grown up! I decided that it was time to settle down and put down some solid roots. So, I bought a house. Not very long after that, I also decided that I was ready for marriage. At long last, I had it all: beautiful kids, a home of my own, a wonderful husband, and a fulfilling job. Life was good.

At forty-five, I was diagnosed with Type 2 Diabetes. I took immediate control of the situation. My father had been diabetic. I'd do anything to avoid the health problems that he suffered with before he passed away. I feared the thought of ever becoming insulin dependent. So, I went on a diet and I stuck to it. I lost sixty pounds between President's Day and Labor Day last year. I did it by eating right and getting lots of exercise, mostly in my flower and vegetable gardens. I looked and felt better than I had in many years. I even impressed myself with my willpower and diligence. It wasn't easy, but I did it!! I was very proud of my accomplishment.

Now, my family and friends will tell you that I am a bit of a hypochondriac. But it's more for comic relief than anything else! I'd never run to the doctor for just any little ache or pain. That'd be too dramatic, even for me! But with my friends, I'd certainly exaggerate any symptoms I might have. For me, a stomach virus was really dysentery. A couple of pimples wouldn't be adult acne. It was an outbreak of smallpox. A headache must be an aneurysm. An allergic rash was surely the first sign of leprosy. An arthritic knee was definitely polio. A mosquito bite would cause me to wail about having malaria. It was an ongoing game. Who could come up with the most horrific disease? Was it silly? Yes! Juvenile? Absolutely! But tons of fun, just the same! And the remedies for all of these terrible ailments were just as amusing to me. Who knew that smallpox could be cured by witch hazel and a cotton puff? Or, that some hydrocortisone cream would eradicate leprosy? Honestly, that was a bit of a disappointment because I was really hoping to get a free trip to the Leper Colony in Hawaii.

On and off for the last couple of years, I'd get a twinge in the left side of my back. Nothing severe. It never lasted very long. It wasn't really a pain. More like an ache. Rather insignificant, I thought. In fact, I never once mentioned it to my doctor. It was so infrequent that I would forget all about it... until it happened again. I chalked it up to being overweight. Naturally, being fat would put a strain on my back! I didn't need my doctor to tell me that I needed to lose weight. I already had a mirror and a bathroom scale. Even after I lost weight, it didn't seem like anything serious. I didn't give it much thought. But now and then, it would come back, just enough to make me reach back and rub my back. And, for dramatic purposes, I'd say to my co-workers "Gee, my kidney tumor is acting up again." It always got a big laugh! Now I wonder if it was a bit of a premonition. Or was it some kind of terrible self fulfilling prophecy? Have you heard the expression, "From your mouth to God's ear?" Well, I wish I had bitten my tongue!

There are certain moments that you never forget. Major life events. I was in the dentist's chair having a root canal the moment the Challenger exploded. The radio was on in the office and the tragedy was announced as I got a shot of Novocain. And, of course we all know exactly where we were and what we were doing the morning of 9/11. I was at work, talking on the phone to a woman in Cape Canaveral Hospital in Florida. I never met her but I even remember her name, Diane. She was watching a morning news program while we tried to work out an insurance claim. I can still hear the sound of her voice when she said, "Oh my God." When something happens that shakes you that hard, to the very core of your existence, you'll never forget even the smallest detail. I now know firsthand that it isn't always a world event that can rock your world with bone jarring intensity. Sometimes it's just a word. Like cancer.

Sunday, September 26, 2004. Exactly one week after my forty-sixth birthday, it was the very last day of my otherwise normal life. By 10:30 that evening I knew in my heart, without any doubt, nothing would ever be the same again. And I was right.

I woke up early that morning. I had to go to the bathroom. I didn't want to jolt myself into staying awake so I kept the light very dim. I just wanted to jump right back under the covers. I noticed a little bit of blood on the tissue and thought I must have gotten my period. I'd been going through perimenopause and my last period was nine months earlier. I thought, "Oh well, glad I didn't toss out those tampons." I put one in and went back to bed thinking I was on the "nine month plan." And frankly, that suited me just fine! For the rest of the day, I checked and rechecked. There was never another drop of blood. I realized I didn't need any more tampons. I decided I was on the new and improved "nine month plan." Three drops of blood and you're finished. "Wow," I thought. This menopause thing is pretty cool. No muss, no fuss!

Later on, after dinner, I had to use the bathroom again. Suddenly I got a very weird feeling. The only way to describe it was that I had a strong urge to urinate, but I just couldn't go. I sat there thinking, "What's up with this?" Finally, after about thirty seconds, which felt more like thirty minutes, that sensation went away. But before I could even get up, something even more bizarre happened. Without warning, something, I didn't know what, just poured out of me. I looked into the toilet and almost fainted. It was full of blood. Quite literally, it was full of blood!! Of course, I immediately panicked. And for a few seconds I just froze in place. I was afraid to move. Afraid if I did, it would happen again.

I didn't know what to do. I didn't want to get up, for fear that I was hemorrhaging. Was I going to bleed to death sitting there? Would whole body parts just fall out of me? I couldn't imagine what was wrong. I just knew that I didn't want anyone to find me that way! Not my family! And I wasn't calling 911 either. I didn't want the police or an EMT! I didn't want an ambulance or even worse, the coroner's van to come! I didn't want anyone to see this. Not anyone! I could imagine the newspaper headlines. I could hear it already, loud and clear "Extra, Extra, read all about it! Local woman dies on the toilet!" Nope! I wasn't having any part of that!

I hoped it was my imagination or some kind of hallucination. But, there was no denying it. It was real. Then, I thought it must be just some freak menopausal thing. Of course! That's what it had to be! What a huge relief! Unfortunately, that idea went right out the window when I realized that the blood wasn't vaginal. I instinctively knew that this was going to be something bad. Something very, very bad. This wasn't something "normal." This wasn't heavy flow from my irregularly scheduled "nine month plan" menstrual cycle. This wasn't good. Not at all!

I opened the bathroom door and I yelled downstairs to my husband who was watching TV with the boys.

I needed to get to the emergency room right away. Now, my family knows that I invent all kinds of medical mysteries, but never once have I asked to go to the hospital. They could hear the seriousness in my voice. There were a few questions along the lines of, "What's wrong?" and "Do you need any help?" But, I wasn't answering anyone's questions. "Just please do exactly what I asked you to do," I said. "And do it NOW!" Then I quickly shut the door.

I didn't want to scare my family. But I most assuredly did not want anyone to come upstairs and see what was actually going on. I just wanted to get out of the house and into the car, preferably, with a minimum of

fuss and bother. So, I carefully and quickly cleaned myself up. And then
I brushed my teeth and ran a brush through my hair. Yes, vanity is my
middle name! When I felt ready, I slowly made my way down the stairs.
I was going in slow motion, but not because I was in any pain. In fact,
nothing hurt at all. I just was afraid to jostle anything around on the
inside. All I could think of was getting away from the kids in case IT
happened again. I was incredulous by the fact that I had no pain.
My family was naturally curious and concerned. One of the boys asked if
I was having a heart attack. The only thing I could tell them was that they
shouldn't worry. I told them that I was just having an issue, and I needed
to get to the ER right away. I said I would call them shortly but right then
and there I just needed to go!! And over my shoulder, as I made my way
to the door, I told them, "Don't worry, it's not a heart attack."

As freaked out as I was on the inside, outwardly I was the picture of
organization and control. I even decided to do the driving. My husband
didn't bother to argue. He just got in and buckled up because he could tell
it was going to be a wild ride. I ran every light and sped down every street
until I got to the closest hospital to our house. It didn't take more
than a few minutes. During the ride, I told Ted what had happened.
I remember him saying, "Don't worry honey. It's probably nothing."
And in my mind I silently answered him, "If that's what you think, then
you have lost your mind."

The ER was empty, and I was glad that I wasn't going to have to wait
long to be seen. I explained my problem to the nurse at the desk and was
immediately taken back to an exam room. My husband had to stay and
do all the insurance paperwork. After getting into a hospital gown I was
asked for a urine specimen. I told the nurse that I really didn't want to pee
ever again. "What if only blood comes out?" She told me not to worry,
that they would take what ever I gave them. To my complete horror, I
filled that cup with nothing but blood. It was terrifying and revolting.
I was mortified to hand it over. I wrapped the cup in wads of toilet paper
and I apologized profusely.

Just a minute or two later, a doctor walked in and asked if I were in
any pain. I said I wasn't. He said I needed a CAT scan. I asked if I were
bleeding to death. He was pretty sure that wasn't the case, but they
needed a scan to find out what was going on. He'd be back after he got
the results. I remember hearing something about a possible urinary tract
infection or a kidney stone. Instinctively, I knew none of those things
were my problem. I've known lots of people who have had UTI's.
No one ever said they almost bled to death in the process. I also knew

that kidney stones cause excruciating pain. I wasn't in any pain at all. I started to cry. I remember telling the nurse that I thought I must have some sort of cancer. Unexplained bleeding like this wasn't going to turn out to be something minor. And because of the speed in which I was being cared for, I knew in my heart that something really bad was going on. I'll never forget that nurse. She patted my hand and didn't say one word. She just looked so sad for me.

That CAT scan was my first. I was amazed at how fast it was over. When I got back to the exam room my husband was waiting for me. I started to cry again when I saw him. He did his best, but there was no comforting me. A few minutes later, the doctor came back in. I could tell by the look on his face that he wasn't about to tell me anything I wanted to hear.

"We need to do another CT scan tomorrow. You're still actively bleeding so we can't send you home tonight. We'll have a urologist come in to see in the morning."

To my husband he said, "It looks like she has a mass in her left kidney."

I wondered why he wasn't speaking to me. So, I piped up, "Excuse me, are you telling my husband that I have cancer?" All I got in response was something to the effect that we'd know more tomorrow. From that non-reply, I already knew the answer. And I was devastated. My world rocked. It was shaking out of control, but only I could see it or feel it.

The first lesson I learned on this journey is that cancer doesn't just affect your health. It touches every aspect of your life. For me, the worst of it has been the pain that my illness causes my family. To hear fear in their voices or to see it in their eyes breaks my heart. I sent Ted home because there was nothing he could do for me, except make me more nervous. The boys needed him at home. I said I'd call the kids to say I was spending the night. I thought they'd worry less. My older son, Dan got the phone on the first ring. The fact that I didn't get a busy signal told me that they were worried. My phone is always tied up! You practically need to make an appointment if you ever want to call us in the evenings. I let him know I was fine, but needed to stay for the night. I assured him again that I hadn't had a heart attack. I told him to tell his brother that I'd see them tomorrow. As he relayed my message, I could hear Matt in the background. He wanted some specifics. I couldn't bring myself to tell him. All I wanted to do was get off the phone before I turned into a blithering idiot.

In the morning a new doctor walked in. He introduced himself as Dr. B., the urologist. A surgeon. In a very grave tone, he said the CAT scan from the night before had shown a "relatively large mass" in my left kidney. I gulped and asked if a "mass" was a synonym for tumor. He just nodded. Do I have cancer? He couldn't say for sure. I needed this second scan. I couldn't get a definitive answer, but it looked very suspicious.

Well, I wanted answers. What was the worst-case scenario? I asked a barrage of questions. Do I need to get rid of this kidney? Obviously there's something wrong with it. I've got two. Is the other one OK? I know people live just fine with just one kidney. Do I need a transplant? Am I on a donor list? Do I need dialysis? Can you go in and rip it out right away? Am I going to die? Do I need a priest? Can we wait until my husband gets here?

It was during my litany of questions that I realized that I didn't like him very much. He didn't answer me. He was cold and robotic. There was nothing at all warm and fuzzy about this guy. So, where's Marcus Welby, M.D., when you need him? But, I brushed away those thoughts and told him to get on with the show. I didn't want to lie there and wait.

It was just after seven o'clock on Monday morning. I called my husband and gave him the news. He was awfully quiet. I asked him to get the boys off to school, call my job and let them know that I needed the day off, and to get up to the hospital right away. Moments later, the orderly showed up with a wheelchair and away we went to Radiology. On the way, he handed me what looked like a loose-leaf binder. I realized it was my "chart" so I opened it and started to read. What jumped out at me were these words: "approximately 7cm tumor." At that point I wanted the world to stop turning so I could jump off. I started to cry. The kid pushing the chair got all upset. Apparently I wasn't supposed to see my own chart. He actually told me he could get in a lot of trouble for even letting me hold it. I thought that was absurd, but I assured him I wouldn't tell anyone and I continued to read it. But by now nothing was registering.

Afterwards, my husband was waiting for me. I told him what I had read in my chart. I could see the worry on his face, but he was very calm and told me that he didn't want me to get all worked up. "Let's wait for the doctor," he said. It seemed to me like there was a whole lot of waiting going on. And I hate to wait.

Finally in came Dr. B with some answers. I had a very large mass in my left kidney. We'd need a pathology report to be sure, but it looked like I had renal cell carcinoma. Speak to me in English, I said. Is it cancer? He said most solid kidney masses are cancer. It was 95% certain. He went on to say that we'd already discussed my willingness to have that kidney removed. At this point he felt that was what we needed to do. He also said he was taking me to the operating room that morning just to find out where the bleeding was coming from. And I was thinking, "Are you a moron?" I haven't been to medical school, but even I knew what was bleeding. My kidney! Of course, I was polite and didn't say any of what I was thinking. But with every passing second I hated this doctor more and more.

Later I was told there had been a blood clot in my bladder. He removed it, and had also done biopsies of my bladder and ureter. He didn't think I was actively bleeding so he was going to "flush" me out. If it was clear I could go home. That didn't seem right! I didn't want to go home with a huge tumor. I wanted him to take it out. Not in a minute. Not in an hour. RIGHT NOW! What was he waiting for? I've watched ER enough times to know that emergency surgery is done all the time. Call NBC! Call Noah Wyle! Call whomever you need to, just get me back to the OR!! STAT!! But, he told me I needed to have several tests, which would be done on an outpatient basis. We'd meet again in his office and discuss the results and go on from there. Calling NBC wasn't an option.

For the next week or so, I took a battery of tests. There was a renal scan to check on both kidneys and to make sure the right one was working well. I had a MRI of my pelvis and abdomen. I had a full body nuclear bone scan. Were they looking for osteoporosis? I was told that when there is suspicion of cancer, they have to check everything. My skeleton was considered another "system." I got scared when the bone scan was over, and they wanted to take X rays of my left knee and my right ankle. Dr. B. ordered X rays of anything that looked suspicious. I couldn't believe that my self diagnosed arthritic knee or trick ankle I got when I was fifteen were considered suspicious! I was also getting really tired of the word "suspicious." I felt like a human science experiment. Everyone either wanted some blood or they wanted to inject me with something radioactive and take pictures.

Once all the testing was done I had an appointment with Dr. B. I got the good news first. The biopsies all came back negative. What a relief! Then he hit me with the bad news. I probably had cancer. "WHAT??" Didn't he just tell me the biopsies were negative? I know I heard him say that! But he hadn't done a biopsy of my kidney. Even without one, he was pretty certain it was cancer.

The surgery wasn't optional anymore. Now it was mandatory. I thought I was going to fall down. I think I actually wanted to fall down! Maybe if I collapsed in a heap on the floor, when I got up I would find out it was all a mistake. He showed me the films on the disc from the tests I had done. I remember thinking they'd be kind of interesting, if they weren't mine. It was a black and white movie of the inside of a human body. Oh look! There were my kidneys. There's the right one. A lovely, perfectly shaped kidney. Then he pointed to the left one. He zoomed in, and my first thought was that it looked more like a misshapen, lumpy potato than anything else. Not even remotely kidney shaped! It most certainly didn't resemble the good kidney on the right side.

I felt like I was seeing and hearing all of this from under water. I wondered if I was having an out of body experience. Nothing seemed real. I had gone to the appointment all by myself in the middle of my workday. In retrospect, that wasn't the best plan I ever had. The words "probably malignant" and "cancer" just played over and over in my head like a broken record. I had no choice but to try to remain calm and rational. I was doing my best to try to memorize every word the doctor said because I still had to go home and replay it all for my husband. Dr. B. called the procedure a left handed radical nephrectomy. "State of the art," he said. He'd make a slit in my belly, put his entire hand inside and take out my offensive kidney. And probably the adrenal gland along with it. And if he bumped into my spleen in the process, he might have to take it out too.

By now tears were running down my face. I did my best to wipe them but they were coming fast and furious. I needed to calm myself down. I needed some levity. I needed a joke. It was the only way to snap out of this nightmare. Nothing can be too awful if you can find somehow to laugh about it. There's a scene in "Steel Magnolias" where Dolly Parton says "Laughter through tears is my favorite emotion." Mine too, I thought. But where was I going to pull a joke out of any of this?

Suddenly I had an idea! I'd worked hard on losing weight before this medical drama. It was an injustice that I could get into such good shape only to find out that I was rotting away on the inside. It was unfair. Shouldn't there be a way to even things up? "Well," I said, "while you're in there taking out my rotten kidney, could you give me a tummy tuck?" Dr. B. looked at me like I had four heads! He didn't even crack a smile. But that didn't stop me. "The insurance company never has to know." At the very least, I expected a smile. Maybe even a snicker. What I got was nothing. No response.

That's when I decided I hated this man. In my mind, his name immediately changed to "Dr. Death." Even to this day, I dislike him intensely. I know it's irrational, but I don't care. He had no sense of humor. Hadn't anyone taught him that laughter is the best medicine?

The rest of the visit went quickly. I wanted to know when I would start the chemo or radiation. Before or after the surgery? Aren't chemo and radiation synonymous with any cancer diagnosis? He told me kidney cancer doesn't get treated with chemo or radiation treatments. It doesn't respond very much to either of them. Surgery is the standard procedure. "We go in and take the kidney out." That was it. Nothing to worry about. You can live just fine with one kidney. No big deal. Four days in the hospital, then six weeks at home in bed to recuperate. A nurse would call me and schedule the pre-op testing and call me with the date. Just like that. End of story. I swear on all that's holy, he acted like the nephrectomy was the answer to all my prayers. Kidney out equals cancer gone. Class dismissed.

The drive home was a blur. I cried the whole way. I remember thinking I was going to have an accident. And that would be a good thing because I'd never have to go home and repeat what I had just been told. Cancer? Oh my God! It was just incomprehensible. How could this be happening? I walked into my house and sank to my knees in front of the kitchen sink. My husband walked in and I started babbling. I was almost incoherent. I was totally inconsolable. Fear, disbelief, anger, rage and pure unadulterated terror consumed me.

Ted didn't know what to do. I almost felt sorry for him. But I was really too busy feeling sorry for myself. He asked me about chemo and radiation and was incredulous when I told him I wouldn't need either of them. Dr. B. said that I was just going to have the kidney taken out and that would be it. It sounded so simple... and too good to be true. But, what did I know?

Well, I might not have had the guts to contradict the doctor, but that didn't stop me from arguing with his nurse. She set my surgery up for the second week of November. I threw a big fit! I wasn't waiting almost a full month! I reminded her that this wasn't a vasectomy or a leaky bladder issue! This was cancer. With a capital C! I said if she was ever unfortunate enough to receive a diagnosis of cancer, she could wait as long as she liked before having it removed. Days, months, even years if she was so inclined. But, I wanted this tumor out of me NOW. Preferably yesterday! But since it was too late for that, tomorrow would be a very good day. I had no intention of sitting around waiting for it to spread. She was just plain mean and told me "that won't happen." All I could think of was that she was the perfect nurse for Dr. B. It was just one more person for me to hate. My only thought was "GET THIS THING OUT OF ME NOW!!" I slammed down the phone and plotted my next move.

Having previously worked in the health care industry, I understand how the system works. I called my family doctor, whom I adore, Dr. R. I cried to her that the urologist was dragging his feet. She agreed. A month was too long to wait. She would call him. Fifteen minutes later, Nurse Nasty called me back. My surgery was moved up two weeks. She made sure to tell me that she had to reschedule and inconvenience other people. Too bad! I told her that bed-wetting, vasectomies, and elderly men with incontinence weren't emergencies. Not to me. This is cancer. It takes top priority. My nephrectomy would be done on October 27, 2004, exactly one month to the day from the initial diagnosis.

During this emotional upheaval, I had to make arrangements at my job. I work for a very small social service agency. I am a housing counselor and do case management for homeless families with children. My job can be stressful, but at the same time it can be very rewarding. My favorite time of year at work is during the winter holidays. We give out Thanksgiving baskets to low income families. It's a huge undertaking and everyone in my department gets very involved in it. We hear a lot of very sad stories from families in need. It has always been my greatest joy at Christmas time to match some of these families with donors who provide wonderful holiday food and gifts for the children. For me, there is nothing better than knowing that kids who would otherwise have a dismal holiday will be showered with clothing and gifts. I was sorry that I was going to miss out on this special time at the agency. I am proud to be associated with a place that does so much for so many.

Now, being a non-profit agency, this isn't a place where one commands a high salary. I was concerned about being out of work so long. I carry the health insurance for my family. The coverage is good but the premiums are high. Even though I only pay a percentage of the cost, my share seems like a fortune. My biggest fear was that I don't have any short-term disability insurance. I had to be out of work for six weeks. I had a couple of weeks of vacation saved, but not much else. If I had to take unpaid medical leave, I wouldn't be able to afford my insurance or my mortgage, let alone anything else. In the end, my fears were relieved. Our executive director took my story to the board of directors. They worked out an arrangement that enabled me to get through that time without worrying. I was able to concentrate on getting well, rather than how to keep afloat. I was given an extraordinary blessing. I will forever be grateful for those who had a hand in making sure that my family was taken care of during that difficult time.

October 27th dawned early. I was scared, but I was prepared. I understood the process. I knew the risks of anesthesia, but I had no fear of any of that. I was a little nervous about how bad it would hurt afterwards. Would I have "phantom" kidney pain? I was told that once I woke up, I would be given as much pain medication as I needed. I planned to ask for the heaviest doses of whatever they had. I was ready!

I was given something to calm me before we left my room. When it came time for my husband to kiss me goodbye, I got nervous. I started to cry, not sobbing or wailing, but tears were freely flowing. A nurse and the anesthesiologist were with me. They were comforting, and the anesthesiologist said he would put a shot into my IV just to calm me down a little bit more. I could feel the drug burning its way up my arm and I noticed a funny taste in my mouth. Then, we were on our way. As they rolled me down the hall, I heard one man say to the other, "Isn't it amazing how quickly that shot makes the tears stop?" I realized that I wasn't crying anymore. I wasn't awake long enough to hear the other man's answer.

When I woke up, my family was in my room. A nurse came in and gave me a shot of morphine, but I was convinced that I had been given a placebo. I was in agony and needed the REAL drugs. She explained that the pain I felt was due to the gas. The gas? What gas? Well, apparently they inflated my belly with gas just prior to the surgery. They literally blew me up like some kind of a balloon! I was told this was a standard procedure. The surgeon needed room to move around and do his job. Well, no one had bothered to warn me about it! So there I was, just horrified to see the belly of a full term pregnant woman attached to ME. It was enormous and incredibly painful. Those gas pains were worse than any labor pains I've ever had!

When Dr. B came in, he said, "I got it all."

I breathed a sigh of relief. The surgery was successful. Painful, but successful. He told me I did great. It had taken four hours but my offending kidney was gone along with my adrenal gland. My spleen was intact. This was all good news. I was elated! He went on to tell me that my cancer was considered Stage III. This was because the tumor had "pooched a little bit" outside of the kidney capsule. Pooched? Hmm... I wasn't familiar with the word. I imagined it to mean something like the way a pimple pushes its way out of your skin. He said that this "pooching" forced them to label it Stage III. I was groggy and asked if "pooched" was a medical term and would he please define it. He lowered his voice and told me the tumor had spread to the fat, which surrounds my kidney. But, he had removed a good deal of the area around my kidney and it had all tested negative for malignancy. The surgery was a complete success. Naturally those were the words I wanted to hear.

There was, however, a problem. I was in excruciating pain. I needed more pain medication. Whatever I was getting didn't work. I needed something stronger. Much stronger! Maybe a double or triple dose! He said he'd order a morphine pump to keep me comfortable, but there wasn't any medicine to make the gas pains go away. Once I started moving around, the gas would begin to work its way out of me. Basically, to get rid of the agony, I needed to walk around and fart! I was just astounded. The morphine made me a little goofy, and must have taken care of most of the surgical pain. I definitely couldn't tell that I had staples in my belly. And there was none of the phantom kidney pain I had dreaded. But, I had gas pains from hell. And, I was caught in a medical catch 22. The pain wouldn't go away until I started moving around, but I wasn't allowed out of bed until the next day. I just couldn't believe this was happening!

This situation was made worse by the fact that I was hungry. I hadn't eaten since the night before the surgery. I was looking forward to dinner. I wasn't thrilled to find out that I couldn't eat until my bowels were moving. Apparently that is part of the problem. Your intestines tend to shut down and "fall asleep" when they are disturbed during a surgical procedure. Moving around makes them "wake up" again. Then the gas passes and the pain goes away.

All it meant to me was that I wasn't allowed to eat. I got nothing but ice chips and a Q-tip looking swab that tasted like mints...YUK... that I was allowed to wet and then swish around in my mouth. I wasn't even allowed to drink a glass of water. I understand the reasoning. Sending food into the digestive system while it's taking some kind of nap is not a good idea. It could back up and cause vomiting. When you have something like twenty-two staples in your stomach, it's not the best time for a bout of vomiting. But still and all, I was famished and the whole thing seemed kind of barbaric to me.

In the morning, the nurse told me I had to get out of bed and start walking. It's the only way to get rid of the gas. I thought she was crazy. I wasn't moving anywhere. I just had my guts ripped out. How could they expect me to start walking around? Well, I did it, but under serious protest. I really just wanted to sleep. I felt like I deserved it. But there I was hobbling through the corridors with both hands holding up my pregnant looking belly and praying that I would fart. And of course, I didn't fart. Not for three days! I walked for miles, down those corridors, in terrible pain and just couldn't pass wind.

In the end they were right, and when the gas finally moved, I was thrilled. The pain immediately lessened. And best of all, now I could eat! I was practically drooling! I was sure I was starving to death. I dreamt of hamburgers and fries. And just my luck, I got a liquid lunch. No food in sight. A cup of tea, a container of milk, some scary green jell-o and a lemon ice. Dinner was more of the same. "Just playing it safe," they told me. I was miserable. I had to wait until the morning, and then I could have a "soft diet." After everything I had been through, my first real meal in four days was going to be cold powdered eggs. Hospital eggs. Yuk!

I was disappointed. But don't you know I polished them off. And I would have begged for more if it weren't for the fact that I was going home! Finally!

It was my understanding from my initial diagnosis and all through my recovery that my biggest long-term concern was going to be about my remaining kidney. Was it in good enough shape to do the entire job for the rest of my life? My plan was, and still is, to live until I am 80. Therefore, this lone kidney has got to last for another thirty-four years. And that means that I really need to take very good care of it.

At my post-op appointment with Dr. B., I asked if I needed to see a nephrologist, a real kidney specialist to keep an eye on my leftover kidney. He said I didn't need to see anyone else. I would see him for frequent visits, and blood work, urine tests, and scans. My right kidney was working perfectly and the bigger issue was to keep a vigilant watch over the spot my old kidney used to occupy. He said there was a slight chance that a tumor might try to grow back in the same place. I asked if I needed to see an oncologist. After all, I had been treated for cancer. He said no, I didn't need one. He reminded me that there was no chemo or radiation for renal cell carcinoma. The treatment is to take it out surgically. We already did that. Other than surgery, there were some biological therapies, mostly experimental, but I didn't need any of that. Just some follow up visits and some scans every 6 months or so. That's it. Thank you and good night.

I didn't feel very comfortable with his plan of action. Or should I say non-action. I'd been treated for cancer. This was important. I wanted to get back to see Dr. R, my family doctor. I've been her patient for many years. She knows and understands me. She also listens to me. By that I mean she really hears me. She validates my concerns. And when she thinks I am wrong, she tells me so. She also laughs at some of my jokes, so I am comfortable with her. I knew that she'd steer me in the right direction. I saw her around Thanksgiving time. She agreed with Dr. B. about the nephrologist. I didn't need one, at least not now. My right kidney was very healthy. All of the tests I would be doing from here on out would tell them if there was any problem. She also told me that I'd be having regular CAT scans just to make sure everything is stable. Then I asked her about an oncologist. She said of course I should see a medical oncologist. I now had a history of cancer. She gave me the name of someone she respected and her office made the appointment for me.

Finally, in December I had gone back to work. I was beginning to feel like myself again. I was getting my strength back. I had been home for exactly six weeks. Four days after I started working again, I went on a business trip to New Orleans with a co-worker. It was wonderful. It was two weeks before Christmas and I felt like I was getting a well deserved gift after going through such an ordeal. I came back from the trip feeling tired, but I had a terrific time.

A week later I had an appointment with the medical oncologist. I remember thinking, "Of all the specialists in the world, this is the last kind I would ever want to have to see." I began to get really creeped out and was becoming depressed. It was a couple of weeks before Christmas and I was having a hard time getting into the spirit of things.

When we met, Dr. E. had a calming effect on me. He had all my pathology reports and operative notes. He had spoken to Dr. B. about my case. He agreed that getting that kidney out of there was the most important thing. He told me that RCC is a relatively rare kind of cancer. He said only about 30,000 people are diagnosed with it each year. Chemo drugs and radiation therapy haven't been too successful in battling this disease. The first line of defense was to remove the kidney. I asked him if I was now in remission. He told me that he wouldn't exactly use that word. But I didn't have to worry because Dr. B. got it all.

Dr. E suggested a consultation with a radiation oncologist. I was confused, because he had just told me that radiation wasn't effective against RCC. He explained that radiation wouldn't be effective if they were trying to shrink a RCC tumor. This was different. He thought I might benefit from radiation to the surgical site. An appointment was made for me to see the radiation oncologist, Dr. MB about a week before Christmas. And I became more depressed.

Luckily, I felt an immediate connection with Dr. MB. The man is a saint. I still consider him my "go to guy." He explained to me why he thought radiation would be a good idea. He said it was kind of a controversial approach to RCC. His explanations made perfect sense to me. Cancer cells are microscopic. There was a possibility that some had gotten away. He thought that radiation at the site of the surgery would kill any RCC cells that might be lurking about. I agreed to go for five weeks of radiation therapy. But, once again I was an emotional basket case. Radiation? It all seemed like a nightmare to me. I was supposed to be "fine."

For five weeks beginning in January, 2005, I went to visit Dr. MB and his staff every weekday morning. I can honestly say that his staff are among the most wonderful people I have ever had the pleasure to meet. I could not believe that I became so attached to them. From the receptionists to the nurses to the technicians, they all made me feel like I was part of their extended family. The treatment actually helped me to ease the depression I was feeling. I finally felt like I was doing something. That helped me emotionally as well. My only real complaint about radiation was that it made me very tired. There were times when it made me nauseated, but Dr. MB gave me something to take that cleared it right up.

I never knew the true meaning of the word fatigue until I had radiation. I still worked full time, and for the most part, unless I felt really sick, I went to work straight from my treatment every morning. As the days wore on, all I really wanted to do was go back to bed, but I just kept plugging along. About a week after my last treatment, in mid February, one morning, I was in the office doing several things at once. My head was swimming with details of a few different clients and I was making copies, taking phones calls, sending faxes, and running back and forth like a mad woman. All of a sudden, I realized I was bouncing back. I had begun to feel more like my real self than I had in a long, long time. I never knew just how draining it was, until it was over.

From then on, I began to feel better and stronger every day. At the end of January I had a CAT scan of my lungs, which had been ordered by Dr. B. They found what they called a "prominent vessel." I didn't know what that meant. Dr. B told me that it could be nothing, just a large blood vessel. He recommended another scan in six months. That seemed like too long to wait. I don't have the patience.

All of my doctors get copies of my reports, so I asked Dr. MB what he thought about the six-month wait. He said it was too long. He suggested another one in six to eight weeks. Dr. MB could ask me to walk through fire and I wouldn't hesitate, so I had another scan in March.

This time there were more "nodules." Now they were in both lungs. Once again he told me that we would check again in six weeks. He indicated that it could be nothing but some inflammation or it could be "something." The thing to do was to keep a close eye on it and see what happens. At this time I was only mildly concerned. I would just do what Dr. MB told me to do.

In May, I had my next scan. Later on in the afternoon, I called his office for the results. It was a Wednesday. The receptionist said she'd leave him a message. On Thursday I still hadn't heard anything, so I called back. I know he's a busy man, so I asked Lisa, the receptionist, to apologize to him for me being such a nag, but I needed to know what the report said. The office staff is just incredibly sweet. She promised to stick a post-it note on his office door. The next morning at eight o'clock Dr. MB called me.

It was Friday, the thirteenth of May. The news wasn't great. He had read the report but wanted to see the actual scan before he called me. He was concerned about the scan. It showed some growth on some nodules and now there were some new ones. What? I went into a tailspin. If I had to get bad news, I wanted it to be from him, but really, I didn't want any bad news. He also told me that there was a problem with the mammogram I had done the same morning as the CAT scan, and I needed to go back for more films. I almost fell down. Something gross is growing in my lungs AND there's something wrong with my breast too? The doctor said he was more concerned about my lungs than whatever it was in my breast and he wanted me to see my medical oncologist, Dr. E. as soon as possible. If I didn't already have an appointment, he would make one for me. I asked if he thought I had lung cancer now. And he told me he didn't think so. I think he said lung cancer would appear differently in the scans. And I know he deals with lung tumors every day, so he knows what he's talking about. I was simply devastated.

By midmorning, I got a call saying I was scheduled to see Dr. E the following Wednesday. That was five days away. I wondered if I was going to live that long. I had been fighting a cold that whole week and now I started coughing. I was certain that the tumors were growing at lightening speed and I would be dead before that appointment ever got here. I also had an appointment set up that week with a pulmonary specialist. It had taken me six weeks to get that appointment. I thought it was a good thing I had asked for it before this last set of scans.

I don't know how I got through work that day or how I made it through the following weekend. I was numb, a zombie, just scared out of my mind. I must have been on auto pilot. Once I got home, I crawled into my bed and stayed there for most of the weekend. All I remember is crying and praying. I didn't want to see anyone or talk to anyone. I just wallowed in misery. I thought if one more person told me "it's probably nothing," I was going to implode! Spontaneously combust! Let the shrapnel poke them in the eye and then they could think THAT was nothing. For me, this WAS something! It was big! I got bad news on Friday the thirteenth. This was just a disaster!!

At some point over that weekend, probably on Sunday, I stopped crying long enough to crawl out of bed. I was still miserable and not in the mood to interact with my family so I turned on the computer. I remembered that in the very beginning of my medical woes how I couldn't find a support group to go to. But, I had gotten lucky and found an online cancer support forum. I didn't really think an online group would be helpful, but I was desperate so I became a member.

I was genuinely amazed at what a nice group of people I had found. They didn't discriminate against me because I didn't have one of the more politically correct cancers. They didn't care that I had kidney cancer. They let me in anyway! In fact, they welcomed me! The social workers that moderate the message boards didn't tell me to find someplace else to go with my unpopular cancer. These people, who I never met in my life, opened their hearts to me. The fact that I had cancer touch my life was enough for them.

I was happy to have finally connected to people who understood how I felt. People who could relate to my feeling all right one minute and falling apart the next. They understood my fears, the changes in my priorities and the changes in my attitude. They clearly understood the effects my cancer has had on my family life and my working life. They let me put all those feelings into words. And most importantly, they made me feel validated. No one seemed to think I was over-reacting. Complete strangers understood the anger I felt about having cancer, the guilt I felt for bringing such sadness to the lives of my husband and children. This group really helped me get through some really tough times. After my radiation treatments were over, I slowly backed away from the group. I didn't need it anymore. As far as I knew, I was fine.

But now, just a couple of months later, I was back. I was at the brink of despair again. So I returned to the forum and posted a long letter. It was almost incoherent, but I was able to release some of the myriad of emotions that were swirling around in me. Writing helps calm me. But in order for it to help me heal, my words require acknowledgement. I don't always feel I can burden my husband or my children with all of my fears. I would be afraid to overwhelm them. And frankly, my family and friends don't always understand what I am going through. It's not their fault. They view it from a different perspective.

But with this group I can vent, rant and rave, or just find a shoulder to cry on. They also understand some of my dark humor. Tumor humor is what I call it. Not everyone in my world is able to handle some of the jokes I make. Some people don't find it funny at all. This online group has also given me the opportunity to step outside of my own personal black cloud, and reach out to people who sometimes are in situations much more serious than mine. It is a good feeling to "give back" and be able to offer them some encouragement and hope. It's wonderful to forget about my own misery while I try to console someone else.

After my long winded, rambling letter I was emotionally drained and I went to bed. I needed to gather some strength so I could go to work in the morning and act like a functioning member of society. The next day during a quiet spell, I checked that website. Among the responses was a note from a woman who told me about a mailing list for people with kidney cancer only. She suggested I subscribe to it. She indicated there was a lot of information out there and that it may be of great help to me. I was a little skeptical, but I decided to check it out. To me, a mailing list is just an invitation for spammers. But, I was just counting down the time until my oncology appointment anyhow. I figured that the doctor was going to hand me a death sentence. What did I have to lose? Deleting all the spam would keep me occupied, right?

Much to my surprise, this mailing list turned out to be the answer to my prayers! I finally found other people with the same disease that I have. They heartily welcomed me to the club that nobody wants to join I didn't have to explain renal cell carcinoma to them. They know all about it. In fact, they explained my disease to me. I have never actually met anyone else who has RCC, but I have finally been able to communicate with people who have RCC or are caregivers of spouses, family members, partners, or friends with this disease. I am not exaggerating when I tell you that these amazing people have given me invaluable information that I so desperately needed.

Within twenty-four hours I had more information about treatment options, as well as the names of kidney cancer specialists, complete with phone numbers, fax numbers, email addresses, and even driving directions! I had a detailed list of the questions I needed to ask my oncologist. And I was given some ideas of what to do if I wasn't able to get the answers I was seeking. Knowledge is power.

I could never explain to you what it was like to walk into my local oncologist's office armed with so much information. I felt like I had an arsenal at my disposal. It was also terrifying to feel that I knew more about my disease than Dr. E. did. I realize that it isn't his fault that he doesn't have any other RCC patients. We are a rare breed. But, since I am his patient, shouldn't he have been doing some research himself? Isn't that his job, as a doctor, to get the information he needs to treat me? If he doesn't know it, shouldn't he be finding it out for me? I guess not.

After a lengthy discussion, with Dr. E, I was horrified to be told that he couldn't make a firm diagnosis as to whether my Stage III cancer had now spread to my lungs. He said my lung nodules, which were obviously multiplying and growing, were still too small to biopsy. The worst news of all was that even if he did a surgical biopsy and found out that it was definitely lung mets, at this time, he would not treat me. I will repeat that, because even now, I find it difficult to understand. Even if he knew for sure that it had spread to my lungs, he would not give me any treatment. Not now. He went on to say that the only available treatments were very harsh and would make me sick. Why give me something that would make me feel sick when right now I am feeling fine? I took that to mean that he wanted to wait until the cancer had gotten so bad that it was making me feel ill...then he would try to treat it. Hmmm. That makes no sense to me.

I walked out of his office and immediately made an appointment with a renal oncologist who was highly recommended by RCC patients from my mailing list. These people know more about this disease than any of my doctors did. It was time to seek a real specialist, someone who works exclusively with kidney cancer patients. I was shocked that I was able to get an appointment within two weeks. It took six weeks to get in to see my local doctors. Can you believe that? Six weeks to see someone who knows nothing about my disease. And only two weeks to see an expert! An expert, I might add, who was a keynote speaker at the American Society of Clinical Oncologists conference this year. Oh, did I neglect to mention that my local oncologist hadn't even heard about the conference? It had taken place only a week prior to my appointment with him. He looked shocked when I spoke about it. Yeah, that made me feel like I was in really good hands! I might as well have gone to the Dog and Cat Clinic!!

I now consider myself one of the lucky ones. I found one of the top experts in the country. Her office is only two states away, just a couple of hours by car. Experts in RCC are relatively few and far between. Most patients have to travel quite a distance in order to be treated by a real specialist in this disease. People fly from all over the country, actually from all over the world, to see what amounts to a handful of real experts. Indeed, I am lucky that I found one of the best almost in my own backyard.

Because there is very little public awareness about renal cell carcinoma, research in the field is extremely under-funded. Right now there are very few FDA approved treatments for this very deadly disease. In a very short period of time, I have been given a wealth of information that my local doctors don't know about or just didn't feel it necessary for me to know. RCC accounts for only about 3% of all cancers diagnosed every year. There are about 30,000 new cases per year and approximately 10,000 RCC patients die every year. This cancer is relatively rare and very aggressive. It is definitely not for the faint hearted!

My new doctor didn't waste a minute changing my diagnosis to Stage IV. The fact of the matter is that there isn't really any time to waste. Although I am not suffering any ill effects at this particular time, the cancer has spread to my lungs. I am about to begin treatment next month. She doesn't feel it's a good idea to wait for my tumor load to be so large that it is causing any complications. The best time to be treated is as early as possible. That makes sense to me!

Although my treatment is FDA approved, the statistics are rather dismal. I am going to be treated with something called High Dose Interleukin 2. This is not exactly chemotherapy. It is considered to be Immunotherapy. I will be given intravenous doses of a protein that is made naturally by the body in very minute amounts. This drug boosts the immune system. It has been found that when RCC patients are given this protein in very high doses, about 7% will be lucky enough to have what is called complete response. In those patients, the disease disappears. The cancer goes into complete remission, hopefully long term. There is approximately the same number of patients, another 7% or so, who will have what is known as a partial response. This means their RCC tumors will either shrink or be shown to stop progressing. These patients may be given the treatment up to three times.

Each treatment consists of five days in the hospital receiving up to fourteen doses of the drug or as many as my body will tolerate before it becomes toxic. Then I will be released for nine days in order to go home and let some of the side effects subside. Then, I will be readmitted to the hospital for five more days to get up to another fourteen doses.

After the second stage of the treatment, I will be released again. I will be given a scan six weeks after the treatment and again at twelve weeks. At that time the situation will be assessed to determine if the treatment had any effect at all. Of course, I am praying to be in that magical 7% who are lucky enough to be told they are NED, which means no evidence of disease. I figure it this way: Somebody has to be in that 7%... why not me? Right?

I realize that the success rate isn't very good... but the fact is that if I do nothing at all there is a better than 99% chance that my disease will continue to spread. And that, of course, means it will kill me. I have no way to know how much time it will take. It is my understanding that RCC is incredibly aggressive. But, so am I. I am going to fight this disease with everything I've got. Then I am going to fight it some more.

Besides the treatment I am about to begin, there really isn't much else out there. That means that no matter how willing I am to fight this disease, at some point I will run out of options. There are only a handful drugs that have shown some promise, but none of them has proven to work for very long. Once they stop working, there isn't much hope.

Without more options, the chances are slim that I will live to a ripe old age. When this dreaded disease entered my life, it robbed me of my sense of security. I find it difficult to keep my composure when my family talks about the future. I always wonder, will I be here next year, or when the boys are old enough to drive? Will I see them in tuxedos on their way to the prom? Will I be there to be burst with pride at their high school graduations? Will I drive them to look at colleges and send care packages to their dorms? Will I get phone calls and letters saying "Please send money?" Will I be able to brag about my son, the doctor or the garbage man or the lawyer or the mechanic? Will I dance with them at their weddings? Will I be there to rock their babies and marvel how much their children resemble the men who were once my own babies? I try not to let them see the true extent of my worry that I may not be there to see some of those things. But my fears are real.

Renal cell carcinoma is the politically incorrect cancer. There is no doubt about it.

And nothing will change until there is public awareness.

CHAPTER 5

Towards Effective Therapy:
Cancer Cell Biology *and* Cancer Research
in Renal Cell Carcinoma
by John A. Copland, Ph.D.

One in three people will develop cancer during his or her lifetime. That translates into an estimated 1.3 million Americans being diagnosed with cancer in 2005 and over 500,000 American dying from cancer in 2005[1]. Worldwide the incidence of new cases per year is around 10 million. To understand carcinogenesis, the process by which normal cells are transformed into cancer cells, we must understand the intricacies of cell function and the molecular pathways that underlie those functions. The cell must be considered in the context of both the organ and the body. The term cancer is used to describe a group of diseases characterized by unregulated cell growth and invasion and spread of these cells from the primary organ to other sites of the body (metastasis). All of these functions of cell growth, invasion and metastasis are regulated by genes within the cancer cell. Sporadic gene mutations caused by environmental factors are responsible for about 95% of all cancers. As many as 50% of those may be preventable. This chapter will begin with a discussion of cancer as a genetic disease followed by a review of renal cell carcinoma (RCC) and its newly recognized susceptibility to chemotherapeutic interventions and conclude with a discussion of ongoing research in renal cell carcinoma including new technologies.

There are over 100 known types of cancers which are classified according to tissue of origin. About 85% of cancers are derived from epithelial cells found in different tissues and are classified as carcinomas. Cancers derived from mesodermal cells such as bone and muscle are called sarcomas and cancers from glandular tissues such as breast are called adenocarcinomas. The tissue of origin gives each cancer its distinguishing characteristic due to the unique set of genes expressed in cells of each tissue as well as the factor(s) causing the cancer such as ultraviolet radiation from the sun for skin cancer and inhalation of cigarette smoke for lung and renal cell carcinoma. Cancer results when the expression of genes is altered in such a manner that cells lose their ability to perform their specialized functions and also take on the following characteristics. These new cancer cells now express genes that promote:

1. cell survival (growth autonomy),
2. evasion of growth inhibitory signals,
3. evasion of cell death
4. unlimited cell replication potential (i.e. immortality),
5. the ability to stimulate the formation of new blood vessels,
6. the ability to invade outside of the organ and metastasize to other organs and
7. inhibition of the immune system (immunosuppression)[2].

Different molecular signaling events regulating these phenotypic events exist in cells. Thus, different combinations of genes are able to control these different processes resulting in cancer cells that are immortal and metastasize to distant organs. The accumulation of these DNA mutations in cells occurs over time and is thought to represent a multi-step process that underlies carcinogenesis (FIGURE 1).

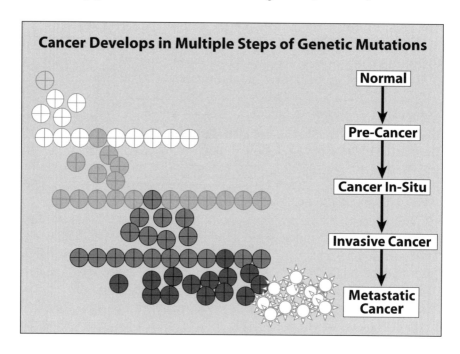

FIGURE 1.   Cancer Develops in Multiple Steps of Genetic Mutations.
Mutations accumulate that result in cancer.

As shown in Figure 1, a normal cell sustains one or more genetic mutation(s) resulting in a pre-cancer cell that continues to replicate its cells. One of the pre-cancer cells sustains one or more genetic mutations leading to a cancer in-situ cell that then continues to replicate. One of the cancer in-situ cells sustains one or more genetic mutations leading to an invasive cancer cell that then continues to replicate and finally more genetic mutation(s) lead to metastatic cancer cells. For these reasons, the stage at which a cancer is diagnosed correlates with outcome. Most people (~95 percent) die of metastatic disease. Individuals diagnosed correctly with cancer in-situ (cancer confined to the organ of origin) that undergo complete removal of the cancer surgically are cured. Also, each cancer is different and individuals with the same cancer do not necessarily have the exact same molecular alterations. More discussion on this topic will follow to assist in your understanding of how each cancer is the same but different. This is why some patients have a good prognosis while others may die from the same cancer. Expression of good genes (tumor suppressor genes) is silenced and bad genes (oncogenes) are turned on enhancing oncogenic activity that results in a shift in homeostasis. Identifying these genes and drugs that are effective against these genes will lead to combinatorial therapy that may cure specific cancers or at least change them to manageable chronic diseases. In summary, adult sporadic cancers are thought to arise from clonal accumulation of multiple genetic alterations, often in a temporal order[3].

Homeostasis is a state of balance, of equilibrium (FIGURE 2). For our purposes, homeostasis is balance between cell birth and cell death. Thus, as an adult, for body homeostasis to be maintained, the same number of cells that divide to create two cells (proliferation) from one must have one cell perish to maintain the same size of our organs and our body.

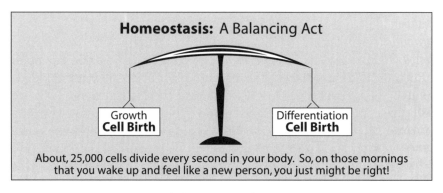

FIGURE 2.   Homeostasis is a balancing act of cell birth and cell death.

An easy to relate to example includes keratinocyte cells that form the outer dermal layer of the skin. Epidermis is the outermost layer of the skin. It consists of two main cell types—keratinocytes and melanocytes—which are produced in the basal layer. The keratinocytes produced in the basal layer migrate upward toward the environment and change their shape to become the protective outer layer called the stratum corneum. This process takes approximately twenty-eight days. The melanoctyes provide the pigment to the skin. Thus, these cells divide, live for a period of time, and die being replaced by new cells to form the outer layer of skin. As shown in FIGURE 3, the process in which a cell replicates itself from one into two daughter cells (proliferation) must be balanced by one cell progressing to a differentiated state to perform the duties of its parent cell while another cell must proceed down a pathway of programmed cell death called apoptosis.

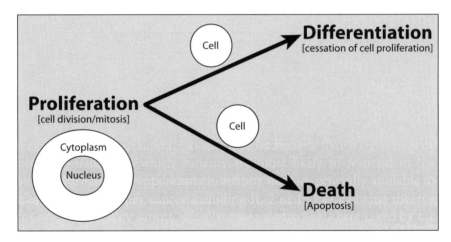

FIGURE 3.   Homeostasis is maintained in the body as cells replicate
                    via cell death and differentiation.

To understand the complexity of any cancer, some basic principles should be understood about the makeup of our body and cancer biology. Our body is organized into cells that have specific functions. Cells are organized into tissues, organs, and blood cells that communicate with one another to perform bodily functions. Each cell has specific functions. For instance, renal proximal tubules' epithelial cells of the kidney are responsible for reabsorption of glucose and sodium as well as secretion of water and urea (a by-product of protein metabolism) into the urine for excretion. Reabsorption is the process of moving solutes from the tubules and returning them to the bloodstream. Both reabsorption and secretion are controlled by the selective permeability of different areas of the renal tubule to water, sodium, and urea and the response of the distal collecting tubules in the kidney. These functions are controlled by molecules or proteins expressed in renal proximal cells. Protein synthesis is regulated by our genes. Our genes are composed of deoxynucleic acids (DNA) and regulatory proteins to form our chromosomes. Thus, as shown in FIGURE 4, genes are transcribed into messenger ribonucleic acids (mRNA) which are then translated into proteins that control the biochemical, molecular, and physiological functions of the proximal tubules. Alterations in levels and functions of key proteins lead to the seven phenotypic changes described earlier and cancer.

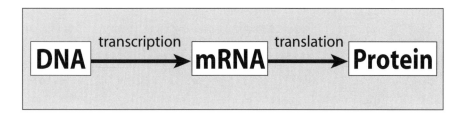

FIGURE 4.   Transcription of DNA into mRNA leads to translation of mRNA into proteins that perform specific functions in a cell.

Transcription is the process whereby DNA is copied resulting in synthesis of mRNA. Thus, DNA acts as the template. Alteration in the DNA template (mutations) or the rate of synthesis of mRNA results in alterations of proteins. mRNA serves as the template for protein synthesis. Transcription of DNA into mRNA occurs in the nucleus of the cell while translation of mRNA into protein occurs outside the nucleus on the ribosomes located in the cytoplasm of the cell.

For any one gene, transcription of DNA into mRNA and translation of mRNA into a protein is an ongoing process. For instance, the regulation of sodium transport in the kidney is important for maintenance of extra-cellular fluid volume and blood pressure regulation. Three different genes encode for three different proteins that regulate sodium transport in the proximal and distal convoluted tubule. They are 1. the type 3 sodium hydrogen exchanger (NHE3), 2. the thick ascending limb of Henle (the bumetanide-sensitive sodium potassium chloride cotransporter (NKCC2), and 3. the thiazide-sensitive sodium chloride cotransporter, (NCC, in distal convoluted tubule) of the kidney[4]. Proteins also have a specific lifespan (half life) and are degraded, thus the need for continual synthesis of new proteins. Many mechanisms are involved in the steps leading to protein synthesis encoded by our genes. Every cell contains the exact same DNA organized into over 25,000 genes which is organized into the twenty-three chromosomes. The organization of the chromatin structure and a class of proteins called transcription factors dictate which genes are expressed in any one cell. This is referred to as epigenetic control. Epigenetic events affect the structure and conformation of chromatin and transcriptional regulation (see FIGURE 4) that lead to changes in expression of a subset of genes in a given cell that result in cancer. Epigenetic alterations in gene expression do not cause a change in the DNA nucleotide sequence and therefore are not mutations. It is this differential gene expression that makes one cell type different from another. Two types of epigenetic mechanisms include histone modifications (acetylation and deacetylation) and DNA methylation (hyper- and hypomethylation). Both of these mechanisms can lead to silencing gene expression. You can envision that the silencing of a tumor suppressor gene by increases in histone deacetylases (deacetylation) and histone methyltransferases (hypermethylation) will enhance carcinogenesis. There is evidence that non-genotoxic carcinogens (agents that do not mutate genes) are epigenetic carcinogens. One such example is phenobarbital[5]. Thus, alterations at the epigenetic level also regulate protein expression and can lead to cancer via alterations in gene expression without mutating DNA[6].

What make each cell unique are the specific sets of approximately 25,000 genes that are expressed in each cell and the level of expression of each gene in the cell. Typically, approximately half or more of the number of total genes available are expressed in any one cell and it is the combinations of genes expressed that determine the functions that each cell will perform. For instance, proximal renal tubules express approximately 17,000 genes, some of which allow these cells to sense and regulate salt, glucose, degraded protein waste and water balance required to maintain body homeostasis. Clear cell RCC originates in the proximal renal tubules' epithelial cells, exemplifying cancer as a genetic disease at the cellular level.

Although cancer is a genetic disease, it is a misconception to think that we are born with genetic defects that cause cancer. These are actually rare events with estimations of about 2 to 5% of cancers being an inherited germ line mutation coming from either of our parents' DNA. As shown in FIGURES 5 and 6, the majority (~ 95%) of cancers are due to events related to our body's interactions with the environment such as smoking, eating certain foods, or exposure to harmful chemicals/radioactivity.

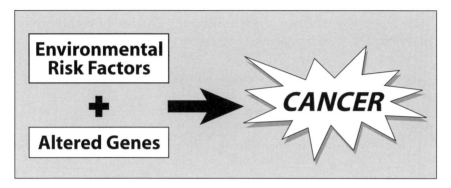

FIGURE 5.   Environmental factors cause cancer by altering genes that cause cancer.

Environmental Causes of Cancer Deaths	
Factor:	Percentage
Tobacco	30%
Diet/Obesity/Sedentary Lifestyle	30%
Occupational/Environmental	7%
Infectious Agents	5%
Alcohol	3%
Ionizing and UV Radiation	2%
Inherited Gene Mutations	2%

FIGURE 6.   Known environmental factors that cause cancer.

These environmental insults can cause DNA damage (carcinogens found in cigarette smoke or ultraviolet radiation from sunlight) or alterations in epigenetic events (histone modification or DNA methylation). The end result is alterations in protein expression regulating molecular events within a cell that lead to the phenotypic or hallmark changes in a cell causing it to become a cancer cell. Again, an epigenetic event is a factor that changes the phenotype through alterations of gene expression (protein synthesis) without changing the genotype. A real example of DNA mutations in RCC is that of dimethylnitrosoamine (DMNA), one of many carcinogens found in cigarette smoke[7]. This chemical in chronic low doses or a single high dose can induce (cause) RCC 100% of the time in rats and mice. Other cancers caused by DMNA include lung and pancreatic cancers in other types of rodents[8]. A mouse given 5 parts per million in drinking water over three months will succumb to RCC. DMNA is an epigenetic event that alters gene expression that then leads to cancer. Smoking is a known risk factor that enhances the chance by at least two-fold of contracting RCC as discussed by Dr. Parker in Chapter 7. If you look back at FIGURE 4, it should become clear that if DNA is damaged then mRNA and in turn protein expression will be vastly altered. Normal cells have mechanisms to protect against DNA damage by way of repairing DNA damage or death via apoptosis. Obviously, these mechanisms are not 100 percent fool-proof since about one-third of chronic smokers contract lung cancer. This is also true for RCC victims who smoke (Chapter 7). Thus, chronic smokers expose themselves directly to a very potent carcinogen via inhalation to the lungs. DMNA then gets into the bloodstream and is exposed to the kidneys and other organs. For lung cancer, smoking is akin to playing Russian roulette with not one but two bullets in a six chamber pistol. Thirty to thirty-five percent of individuals who are diagnosed with RCC are also chronic smokers.

   To summarize to this point, you now should have an understanding of the complexity in the organization and functions of cells within a tissue or organ and the complexity of all organs and tissues within the body. You should understand that cancer is a genetic disease in which alterations in gene expression either through DNA mutation or epigenetic events alter protein expression critical to cell function. Not one but many proteins that regulate cell survival, renewal, death, mobility, immunity, and invasiveness must be altered for cancer to occur. Think of the number of events occurring every second within a cell and your body! With the completion of sequencing the human genome in 2003, it is now thought that humans contain about 25,000 genes in each one of our cells.   The synthesis of mRNA and translation into proteins are occurring constantly.   It is also estimated that our bodies are each composed of 10^{14} or 100,000,000,000,000 cells. Think again of all of these events that are occurring in each cell and then multiply that by 10^{14} cells. I am ceaselessly amazed by the miracle of life and the exquisite biochemical and molecular events that allow our bodies to maintain homeostasis as we experience life.

   Over the past year (2004-2005), clinical trials are now demonstrating that RCC once thought to be chemoresistant is not (Chapter 3,

Dr. Jaimie Merchan). Thus, a new era has dawned yielding hope and expectations that one day in the near future effective therapies leading to longevity and good quality of life will result from new drugs being developed and brought forward into clinical trials for RCC patients. It is my belief that effective combinatorial therapy will be discovered as aberrant signaling pathways are identified in RCC. Much work remains to be done in basic research, translational research, drug discovery, and clinical trials. New technologies combined with old are leading scientists and physicians to new discoveries into the molecular characterization and mechanisms regulating RCC tumor formation (carcinogenesis) and tumor progression to metastasis. Understanding these molecular mechanisms will allow for a rational plan to design molecular targeted drugs that will be effective against any cancer including RCC. The sequencing of the human genome and identification of mRNAs in humans have allowed for the development of genomic technologies (reviewed in [9]).

One such new technology is genomics or gene array analysis which allows for the analysis of the expression of all genes from a tissue or cancer. Thus, mRNA levels from RCC tissue can be compared to normal kidney tissues to identify altered genes in RCC[10-15]. Identification of key genes regulating RCC can be revealed and drugs developed to target inactivation (oncogenes) or activation (tumor suppressor genes) of genes and their gene products (proteins). One could envision the future using a rationale design based upon molecular profiling to treat a cancer patient with combinations of drugs inactivating key signaling pathways necessary for cancer cell survival. The newfound responsiveness to treatment is a result of new drugs that target specific molecules found to be over expressed in RCC tissues (see Chapter 3, antagonists to epidermal growth factor/EGF and vascular endothelial growth factor/VEGF signaling). These novel molecular targeted therapies are now demonstrating efficacy in RCC clinical trials.

Clinical applications using genomics (as well as proteomics, an evolving technology) include disease diagnosis, disease classification, disease prognosis, predicting drug toxicity, identification of new molecular drug targets, and outlining treatment strategies based upon molecular targets that are druggable as illustrated in FIGURE 7. Some successes in RCC include disease classification,[13, 14, 15] disease prognosis,[16] disease diagnosis[17] and novel drug targets[6, 12].

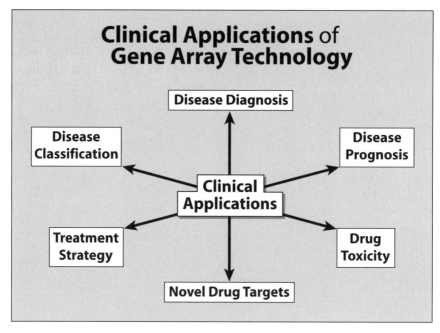

FIGURE 7.   Cartoon of clinical applications using gene array technologies.

To reiterate, when a kidney is removed from a patient undergoing surgery for a renal mass, RNA is isolated from the tissues and mRNA from adjacent normal tissue is compared to that of RCC tissue. Changes in mRNA expression of the altered genes can then be analyzed to identify a molecular profile characteristic of RCC. Using genomic technology combined with bioinformatics (statistical analysis of large biological data files), hundreds of genes in a single assay can be identified as being altered in RCC. In the dendogram (or heatmap) shown in FIGURE 7, hundreds of genes are identified to be consistently different in six patients diagnosed with early stage localized clear cell RCC when compared to patient-matched normal tissue mRNA levels. Red represents genes that are expressed at high levels while green represents genes that are expressed at low levels. Black represents expression between high and low levels. Each row represents a gene and each column represents the patient's normal or tumor tissue. A biostatistical analysis technique called hierarchical clustering groups genes according to their similarity in expression levels. Thus, the first six columns represent the mRNA expression of tumor tissues and the last six columns represent mRNA expression levels of normal tissues. In the top half of the dendogram, you can easily see that 305 genes are elevated (red) in RCC tissue as compared to patient matched normal renal tissue (green). In the bottom half of the dendogram, you see the opposite or the loss of expression of 560 genes (green) in RCC patients compared to that of normal renal tissue (FIGURE 8). Think about this: 865 genes have changed in an early stage, localized RCC tumor from that of its normal tissue counterpart. This exemplifies the astounding complexity of cancer and the complexity of effecting a cure or the ability to downgrade cancer to that of a chronic disease as opposed to a potential death sentence. At first blush, one would believe that RCC is incurable.

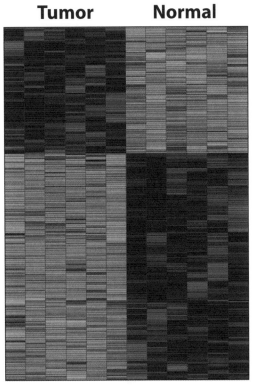

Tumor   Normal

FIGURE 8.   Dendogram demonstrating genes that are expressed differently between normal kidney tissue and RCC from patient samples. Red indicates hot or upregulated genes and green indicates cool or down-regulated genes. Each row represents a gene and each column represents mRNA expression levels from either tumor or normal tissue. Hierarchal clustering has identified genes that are expressed at similar levels in RCC patient tissues (Tumor) compared to that of normal tissue. A set of 305 genes are elevated in tumor tissue (red, top half of dendogram) while 560 genes are suppressed in tumor tissue (green) compared to normal tissue (bottom half of dendogram).

How does one organize and interpret this data to understand molecular mechanisms of carcinogenesis? Can this disease really be cured with hundreds of genes being altered? The answer is yes. Like our society, this is a hierarchal system in which master genes exist that control many other genes. Thus, by altering the expression of a master gene, up to hundreds of genes can be corrected. So, there is potential that a handful of molecular targeted drugs will lead to effective therapies. The question remains for all cancers which ones and how many? In FIGURE 9, some examples of molecular signaling pathways are shown to illustrate the point that one altered gene can lead to alteration of many genes leading to phenotypic changes such as cell proliferation to promote a cancer. In FIGURE 9, top left signaling pathway, follow the EGFR or epidermal growth factor receptor signaling pathway through Ras, Raf, MEK, ERK, E2F. Activation of this signaling pathway leads to cell replication or proliferation. EGFR is one of many cell membrane proteins that promote cell proliferation but it specifically binds tumor secreted and blood circulating EGF and TGFα (transforming growth factor alpha). TGFα is up-regulated in RCC and it is secreted from tumor cells. Secreted TGFα can then bind to the cell surface portion of EGFR to stimulate this signaling pathway that then alters a set of genes that enhance

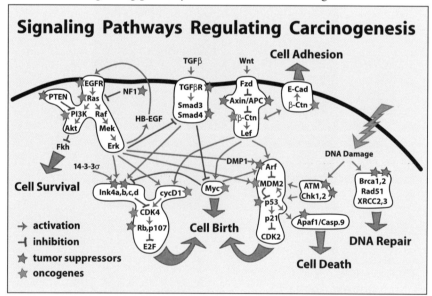

FIGURE 9.   Molecular signaling pathways that regulate cell survival, proliferation, and death (apoptosis). Genes with orange stars when overexpressed act as oncogenes while genes with green stars act as tumor suppressor genes and their protein expression when suppressed promotes cancer. (Adapted from[18])

cell proliferation. You can begin to envision that when one gene, such as TGFα, is altered, it can set off a whole set of other genes that then enhance cell growth. In grouping genes from the genomic data (dendogram), we can begin to identify oncogenic signaling pathways that can be targeted for drug therapy. Note many oncogenes and tumor suppressors remain to be discovered. Clearly, many altered signaling pathways contribute to RCC as shown by the changes in 865 genes in the dendogram in FIGURE 8. One could also envision, in the not too distant future, personalized medicine in which a biopsy is performed to identify genes that must be altered to effect a cure or down-grade cancer to a chronic disease. So, for a patient diagnosed with cancer, selected combinatorial therapy would be personalized for each patient based upon molecular alterations in genes (and/or proteins) expressed in that person's cancer (FIGURE 10). The technologies to be used to identify global changes in a patient's cancer most likely will involve many technologies that may include genomics, proteomics and other technologies not mentioned in this chapter.

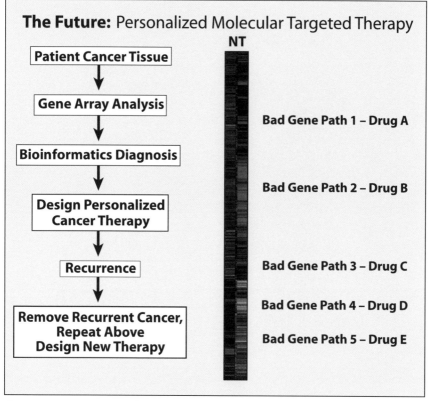

FIGURE 10.   A vision of the future for treating diseases such as cancer.

The future is one of optimism. We have the technologies and a knowledge base to build upon and to effect changes in cancer treatment. Our work now is to identify and verify the critical genes that can be targeted for therapy and to develop drugs or other therapeutics. These must then be tested and verified in preclinical models and finally in clinical trials.

The road ahead is much clearer to effect change in the lives of individuals diagnosed with RCC. Through development of molecular understanding of tumor formation and tumor progression, we are marching toward new therapeutics that will revolutionize the treatment of renal cell carcinoma.

NOTES:

NOTES:

CHAPTER 6

Pathological Features *of* Renal Cell Carcinoma *and* Their Impact *on* Patient Survival
by John C. Cheville, M.D.

INTRODUCTION

There are various types of cancer that can arise in the kidneys; however, over 90% of kidney cancers among adults are classified as renal cell carcinoma (RCC). There is considerable variability in survival for patients with RCC based on a number of pathologic features (i.e., structural features of the tumor determined upon microscopic examination by a pathologist). Herein, pathologic features important in predicting survival for patients with RCC are reviewed including subtype, sarcomatoid differentiation, the TNM classification, tumor size, tumor grade, and tumor necrosis. Throughout, the distributions of these pathologic features are summarized using data from 3,001 patients in the Mayo Clinic Nephrectomy Registry. This Registry contains pathologic features and long-term follow-up for all patients treated surgically for RCC at Mayo Clinic Rochester since 1970.

IMPACT ON PATIENT SURVIVAL

The impact of various pathologic features on survival is illustrated using Kaplan-Meier plots. The Kaplan-Meier method is commonly used to estimate the survival of a group of patients starting at a specific point in time, in this case surgery for RCC, and ending at a specific point in time, in this case death from RCC. The horizontal axis on the plot is time from surgery while the vertical axis is the cancer-specific survival percentage. At time 0 on the plot all patients are still alive and consequently the estimated cancer-specific survival rate is 100%. Over time, however, patients die from their disease and the estimated cancer-specific survival rate falls. If we were able to follow every patient until they died we would be able to estimate survival rates at specific points in time as simply the number of patients still alive divided by the total number of patients in the group. However, we typically can not wait to estimate survival rates until every patient has died. Furthermore, a few patients may be "lost to follow-up" if they do not return to Mayo Clinic for their follow-up care and do not respond to follow-up questionnaires regarding their disease status. These patients are "censored" at the point in time when we last knew they were alive. Even though their data are incomplete, these patients provide important information with which to estimate survival rates up until the point in time when they are censored. The Kaplan-Meier method is one method that can be used to estimate survival rates in the presence of censoring and will be used to illustrate how various pathologic features impact survival throughout the rest of this chapter.

PATHOLOGICAL FEATURES

SUBTYPE

In 1997, an international consensus conference on RCC sponsored by the Union Internationale Contre le Cancer (UICC) and the American Joint Committee on Cancer (AJCC) outlined an accepted classification system for the subtypes of RCC. The UICC/AJCC adopted the classification system originally proposed at the Heidelberg conference in 1996. The participants at both conferences proposed that RCC be classified as clear cell, papillary, chromophobe, or collecting duct. In addition, RCC that does not fall into one of these four groups is classified as RCC, not otherwise specified. This classification recognizes that RCC consists of several subtypes with distinct pathologic and genetic characteristics. The most common subtype is clear cell RCC, followed by papillary and chromophobe RCC. The distribution of subtype for patients in the Mayo Clinic Nephrectomy Registry is summarized in TABLE 1.

TABLE 1: Distribution of RCC Subtypes

Clear Cell	2,424 (81%)
Papillary	409 (14%)
Chromophobe	141 (5%)
Collecting Duct	7 (<1%)
Not Otherwise Specified	20 (<1%)

There are significant differences in patient outcome by RCC subtype. The cancer-specific survival rates at five years following surgery for patients with clear cell, papillary, and chromophobe RCC are 72%, 91%, and 87%, respectively (FIGURE 1). Patients with clear cell RCC have a worse prognosis compared with patients with papillary and chromophobe RCC.

However, a small proportion (approximately 4%) of patients with clear cell RCC have a variant called cystic clear cell RCC. Cystic clear cell RCC is typically cured by surgery alone. In fact, no patient in the Mayo Clinic Nephrectomy Registry has died from cystic clear cell RCC.

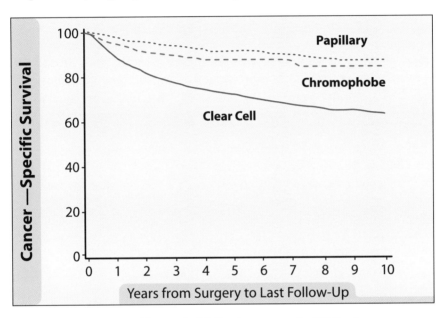

FIGURE 1:   Cancer-specific survival following surgery by RCC subtype.

SARCOMATOID DIFFERENTIATION
    Sarcomatoid differentiation is a high-grade area within a RCC tumor that contains large and irregularly shaped cells. In the past, sarcomatoid RCC was considered a unique subtype; however, it was dropped from the 1997 UICC/AJCC and Heidelberg classification since sarcomatoid differentiation can be found in all of the RCC subtypes. The presence of sarcomatoid differentiation is rare; only 5% of clear cell RCC tumors in the Mayo Clinic Nephrectomy Registry have this feature. Although rare, sarcomatoid differentiation is associated with a very poor prognosis for all subtypes of RCC. The cancer-specific survival rates at five years following surgery for patients with and without sarcomatoid differentiation are 12% and 75%, respectively.

TNM CLASSIFICATION
    The primary tumor (T), regional lymph nodes (N), and distant metastases (M) classification for RCC is summarized in TABLE 2. The

TNM classification describes the stage and extent of disease, from a tumor that is confined to the kidney to a tumor that spreads beyond the kidney. The classification standardizes the description of a tumor, improves communication between pathologists and clinicians, and guides post-operative follow-up. Each component of the classification is described in greater detail in the following three sections.

The TNM classification has been recognized as an excellent prognostic factor for patients with RCC since its introduction in 1978, although it continues to be modified, most recently in 2002. For simplification, the TNM classification can be collapsed into four stage groupings (TABLE 2). Among patients with clear cell RCC at Mayo, there are 1,147 (47%) patients with stage I disease, 370 (15%) with stage II, 512 (21%) with stage III, and 395 (16%) with stage IV disease. The association of the TNM stage groupings with cancer-specific survival for these patients is illustrated in FIGURE 2. The cancer-specific survival rates at five years following surgery for patients with stage I, II, III, and IV RCC are 95%, 81%, 58%, and 14%, respectively.

TABLE 2: 2002 TNM Classification and Stage Groupings for RCC

T	Primary Tumor
TX	Primary tumor cannot be assessed
T0	No evidence of primary tumor
T1a	Tumor 4.0 cm or less in greatest dimension, limited to the kidney
T1b	Tumor more than 4.0 cm but 7.0 cm or less in greatest dimension, limited to the kidney
T2	Tumor more than 7.0 cm in greatest dimension, limited to the kidney
T3a	Tumor invades adrenal gland or perinephric tissues but not beyond Gerota's fascia
T3b	Tumor grossly extends into renal vein(s) or vena cava below diaphragm
T3c	Tumor grossly extends into vena cava above diaphragm
T4	Tumor invades beyond Gerota's fascia
N	Regional Lymph Nodes
NX	Regional lymph nodes cannot be assessed
N0	No regional lymph node metastases
N1	Metastases in a single regional lymph node
N2	Metastases in more than one regional lymph node
M	Distant Metastases
MX	Distant metastases cannot be assessed
M0	No distant metastases
M1	Distant metastases

Stage Groupings	T	N	M
I	T1	N0	M0
II	T2	N0	M0
III	T1	N1	M0
	T2	N1	M0
	T3	N0, N1	M0
IV	T4	N0, N1	M0
	Any T	N2	M0
	Any T	Any N	M1

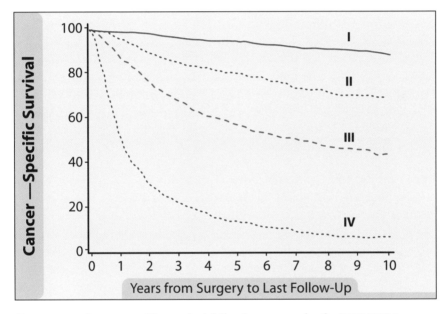

FIGURE 2:   Cancer-specific survival following surgery by the 2002 TNM
            stage groupings for patients with clear cell RCC.

PRIMARY TUMOR (T)

The T1a, T1b, and T2 classifications are reserved for tumors that are confined to the kidney. A tumor is classified as T1a if it is four centimeters (cm) or less; T1b if it is more than four cm but not more than seven cm; and T2 if it is more than seven cm. In addition to tumor size, another measure of the anatomical extent of the tumor is involvement of the ipsilateral adrenal gland. The adrenal glands, part of the body's endocrine system, are located directly above each kidney. Renal cell carcinoma can invade the adrenal gland though direct extension from the primary tumor or through metastases (i.e., tumor that spreads through the lymphatic system or the blood vessels). Direct extension is defined as contiguous spread of the tumor through the peripheral perinephric fat into the ipsilateral adrenal gland. Metastatic involvement is characterized as a discrete nodule of RCC within the ipsilateral adrenal gland with uninvolved intervening perinephric fat between the adrenal gland and primary tumor. While metastatic involvement is classified as M1, direct extension is currently classified as T3a along with tumors that invade the perinephric or renal sinus fat. The 2002 primary tumor classification also recognizes the importance of tumor extension into the renal vein or inferior vena cava and classifies these tumors as T3b or T3c. Extension of the tumor beyond Gerota's fascia, a thin membrane that surrounds the kidney and perinephric fat, is classified as T4. Among patients with clear cell RCC in the Mayo Clinic Nephrectomy Registry, there are 628 (26%) patients with T1a disease, 586 (24%) with T1b, 466 (19%) with T2, 220 (9%) with T3a, 475 (20%) with T3b, 19 (1%) with T3c, and 30 (1%) with T4 disease. The cancer-specific survival rates at five years following surgery for patients with T1a, T1b, T2, T3a, T3b, T3c, and T4 disease are 96%, 85%, 67%, 47%, 44%, 37%, and 14%, respectively.

REGIONAL LYMPH NODES (N)

The 2002 regional lymph node classification for RCC is based on the number of positive hilar, abdominal paraaortic, and paracaval lymph nodes identified during surgery. The NX classification indicates that no regional lymph nodes were removed during surgery; N0 indicates that one or more regional lymph nodes were removed, but none contained metastases; N1 indicates the presence of metastases in a single regional lymph node; and N2 indicates the presence of metastases in more than one regional lymph node. The presence of metastases in the regional lymph nodes is rare; only 5% of patients with clear cell RCC in the Mayo Clinic Nephrectomy Registry are N1 or N2. However, this feature is associated with a very poor prognosis. The cancer-specific survival rates at five years following surgery for patients with and without regional lymph node metastases are 18% and 75%, respectively.

DISTANT METASTASES (M)

Distant metastatic disease at the time of surgery portends a poor prognosis for all subtypes of RCC. Among patients treated surgically for clear cell RCC at Mayo Clinic, 15% present with disease that has metastasized to other organs of the body. The cancer-specific survival rates at five years following surgery for patients with and without distant metastases are 14% and 82%, respectively.

TUMOR SIZE

Although tumor size is incorporated into the TNM classification, studies from Mayo Clinic have shown that size is an important prognostic feature for patients treated surgically for RCC even after accounting for the TNM classification. Studies from our institution have also demonstrated that as the size of a RCC tumor increases the likelihood that it is clear cell and high-grade (i.e., grade 3 or 4) increases. For example, among patients with tumors less than five cm in the Mayo Clinic Nephrectomy Registry, 76% have clear cell and 20% have papillary RCC. In contrast, among patients with tumors 10 cm or greater, 84% have clear cell while only 8% have papillary RCC. Among patients with clear cell RCC, only 20% of those with tumors less than five cm are high-grade compared with 76% of those with tumors 10 cm or greater.

TUMOR GRADE

Several grading systems for RCC have been proposed, all demonstrating an association with patient outcome, but there is no international consensus regarding which grading system should be used. Currently, the most commonly employed system is referred to as the Fuhrman grade. The Fuhrman grade is based on nuclear size and shape and the prominence of nucleoli. (Nucleoli are small structures within the nuclei that are involved in cell division.) At Mayo Clinic, a grading system modeled after Fuhrman's criteria is used. Grade 1 tumors have small, round nuclei with inconspicuous nucleoli visible only at high magnification, as seen under a microscope. Grade 2 tumors contain round to slightly irregular nuclei with mildly enlarged nucleoli visible at intermediate magnification. Grade 3 tumors have round to irregular nuclei with prominent nucleoli visible at low magnification, while grade 4 tumors contain enlarged cells of many different shapes. The distribution of tumor grade by subtype for patients in the Mayo Clinic Nephrectomy Registry is summarized in TABLE 3.

TABLE 3: Distribution of Tumor Grade by RCC Subtype

	Clear Cell N=2,424	Papillary N=409	Chromophobe N=141
Tumor Grade			
1	262 (11%)	8 (2%)	2 (1%)
2	1,051 (43%)	250 (61%)	92 (65%)
3	907 (37%)	145 (35%)	33 (23%)
4	204 (8%)	6 (1%)	14 (10%)

Tumor grade is significantly associated with patient outcome, even after accounting for other important prognostic features. The association of tumor grade with cancer-specific survival for patients with clear cell RCC is shown in FIGURE 3. The cancer-specific survival rates at five years following surgery for patients with grade 1, 2, 3, and 4 clear cell RCC are 95%, 90%, 56%, and 18%, respectively. Although patients with grade 2 tumors are more likely to die from RCC compared with patients with grade 1 tumors, this difference is not statistically significant. Other studies that have used the Fuhrman grading system have reported similar results. These findings suggest that a three-tiered grading system may be appropriate for RCC. However, use of a three-tiered grading system without strict adherence to standardized criteria would likely result in an increase in the frequency of grade 2 tumors and lessen the ability of grade to predict clinically important outcomes.

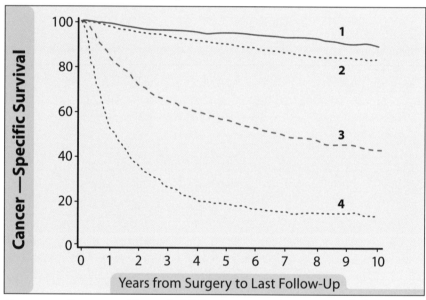

FIGURE 3:   Cancer-specific survival following surgery by tumor grade for patients with clear cell RCC.

TUMOR NECROSIS

Tumor necrosis in RCC is characterized by sheets of degenerating and dead cells. The cause of tumor necrosis is not entirely known, but it may occur when cells outgrow their blood supply. The impact of tumor necrosis on patient outcome varies considerably by subtype. Although patients with papillary RCC at Mayo are more likely to have necrotic tumors (46%) compared with patients with clear cell RCC (29%), the finding of necrosis in a papillary tumor is not significantly associated with cancer-specific survival (FIGURE 4). In contrast, the finding of tumor necrosis in clear cell RCC is indicative of aggressive tumor behavior (FIGURE 5).

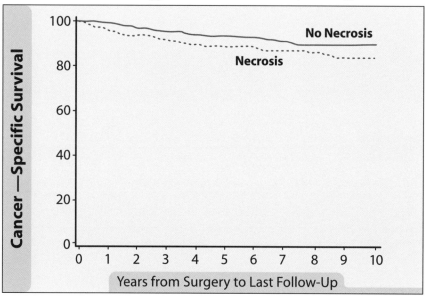

FIGURE 4:   Cancer-specific survival following surgery by tumor necrosis for patients with papillary RCC.

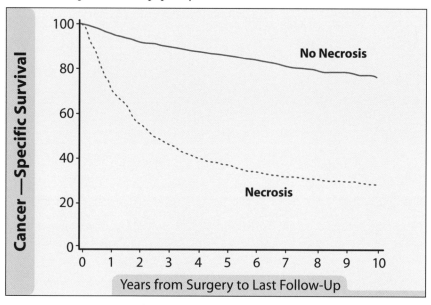

FIGURE 5:   Cancer-specific survival following surgery by tumor necrosis for patients with clear cell RCC.

Conclusion

Accurate subtyping of RCC is critically important and should be done as part of routine pathological evaluation. The TNM classification, already a powerful prognostic feature, will continue to evolve. This review also highlights the importance of assigning a tumor grade based on standardized and reproducible criteria. Lastly, it is increasingly evident that tumor necrosis and sarcomatoid differentiation are compelling prognostic factors, on par with tumor grade, and should be routinely assessed.

NOTES:

CHAPTER 7
Renal Cell Carcinoma Epidemiology
by Alex Parker, Ph.D.

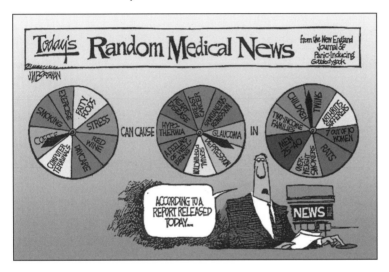

INTRODUCTION

Unfortunately, in the world of cancer research, the sentiment expressed in the above cartoon is not that far from the truth. Indeed, the scientific and medical communities constantly bombard the general public with messages and warnings about certain lifestyle and dietary choices that may increase their risk of developing cancer. Perhaps even more troublesome than the sheer volume of this information is the fact that these well-intentioned messages are often inconsistent, confusing and sometimes even in direct conflict with one another. We've all seen this unfortunate scenario play out in the media. One week a study comes out claiming that drinking orange juice will lower your chances of developing a particular cancer. Then later that same year, a second study will claim with equal certainty that the consumption of orange juice has no bearing whatsoever on whether or not a person will develop cancer. Given these mixed messages, it is not surprising at all to find that many people are frustrated with the research community's inability to provide a clear and consistent message about what causes cancer. In the chapter that follows, my goal is to try to provide some clarity to the seemingly blurred issue of what puts a person at risk of developing renal cell carcinoma (RCC). As a cancer epidemiologist with a particular interest in urologic cancers, a large portion of my research focuses on studying the distribution and determinates of RCC. Put another way, I spend a lot of my time trying to answer the *"when, where and why"* of RCC. Now all hubris aside, I certainly don't profess to have a patent on the truth about RCC, but hopefully in the paragraphs that follow I can provide a roadmap to help the reader navigate the often murky waters of RCC epidemiology.

GAUGING THE IMPACT OF RENAL CELL CARCINOMA

A logical place to start this discussion is to take a look at some standard descriptive statistics that will put RCC into perspective and help us to get an idea of the burden this cancer places on our society. Basically, before we begin talking about what may or may not cause RCC and what we can do to avoid it, we first need to orient ourselves to the depth of this disease and get a better understanding of its overall impact on public health. Now any good discussion of RCC should certainly lead off by providing some clarification with regard to the current terminology. The term 'kidney cancer' is generally used to refer to any cancer that arises in the kidney. Luckily for our discussion in this chapter, the vast majority of cancers diagnosed in the adult kidney (around 85-90%) are classified as RCC. However, if the terminology issues ended there life would be simple, but to my knowledge no one has ever claimed life to be simple. Therefore, we are forced to further refine our definition a bit more. The term "RCC" actually refers to a collection of tumors for which there are currently four widely recognized subcategories: clear cell RCC, papillary RCC, chromophobe RCC and collecting duct RCC (Lohse, 2005). Again, much to our pleasure, we are lucky that the vast majority of RCC tumors fall into the clear cell category (about 85%). So just remember two points as we continue this discussion on descriptive statistics: (1) the vast majority of kidney cancers are classified as RCC and (2) the large majority of those RCCs are of the clear cell variety. I apologize for starting out with such a seemingly monotonous clarification but with these terminology issues taken care of, we are now free to press on with our initial discussion of the impact of RCC on our society.

RCC INCIDENCE

Quantifying the burden of any disease in a particular population is a difficult task. We must be mindful that no single measure can effectively capture all of the multi-dimensional aspects of RCC and how it relates to individuals, the health care system and society at large. But we have to start somewhere, right? In 2005, the American Cancer Society estimates that there will be approximately 36,000 new cases of RCC diagnosed in the United States (Jemal, 2005). To add some perspective to that number, those 36,000 cases of RCC will translate to approximately 3% of all new cancer cases diagnosed in 2005. Looking at it that way, one might conclude that RCC is a relatively rare cancer; and in truth, they'd be right. But as we all know, numbers sometimes don't tell the whole story. For that reason, we really should look a little closer. A common statistic used to measure disease burden and better gauge the impact of a disease on a population is the *incidence rate* of the disease, defined simply as the number of new cases diagnosed in a defined number of people (usually per 100,000 individuals) for a given time period[i]. Overall, the incidence rate for RCC in the U.S. is about 12 cases per 100,000 individuals (for reference, compare that with breast cancer at 73 cases per 100,000 and prostate cancer at 76 cases per 100,000) (Reis, 2005). Again, given that the incidence rates are about six times higher for breast and prostate cancer, we might conclude by looking at these numbers that RCC pales in comparison to these "bigger players". However, we still need to withhold judgment until all the facts are in. Suffice to say, incidence rates still only reveal part of the picture, as we will see a bit later.

While they certainly don't provide the whole story, the real utility of looking at incidence rates is that they allow us to make comparisons across important subgroups of individuals and thereby learn more about the true impact of this disease. For instance, the incidence rate of RCC is about twice as high in men (16 cases per 100,000) as it is in women (8 cases per 100,000) (Reis, 2005). Similarly, if we compare across categories of race/ethnicity we find that RCC incidence is highest among African Americans (14 cases per 100,000) and Caucasians (12 cases per 100,000), slightly lower among Hispanics (11 cases per 100,000) and Native Americans (10 cases per 100,000) and lowest among Asians and Pacific Islanders (6 cases per 100,000) (Reis, 2005). From a more global perspective, the incidence of RCC is highest in developed countries and shows considerable variability when you compare across different geographic regions. For example, incidence rates for RCC are highest in North America, Northern Europe, Eastern Europe and Australia while rates are considerably lower in Asia, Africa and the Pacific (reviewed in Linbald and Adami, 2002). So to this point, just by looking within some broad, general subgroups (i.e. gender, race, geographic region) we begin to see that there is quite a bit of variation in the impact that this cancer has on different populations. What's more, as some of you may have already guessed, this same variation can provide vital clues to help us uncover some of the lifestyle and dietary factors that can increase the risk of developing RCC...but more on that later.

So far, we've used incidence rates to look at some important categories that tell us a little bit about *where* RCC occurs (i.e. incidence is higher in men, African Americans, North America etc.). Now it's time to focus attention on the *when*. FIGURE 1 depicts the incidence rates for RCC (shown along the vertical axis) by increasing age (shown along the horizontal axis). The rates for men (■—■), women (◆—◆) and both genders combined (●—●) are all provide on this one graph.

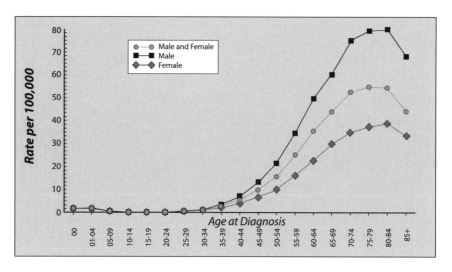

FIGURE 1:   Incidence Rates for RCC Across Age Groups
            This graph shows the incidence rates for men (■—■), women
            (◆—◆) and both genders combined (●—●). Clearly, RCC is an
            extremely rare cancer before the age of 35 and after that the incidence
            rises sharply to a peak at around age 75. We also note from this graph
            that the incidence of RCC is generally higher among males than females.

Ries LAG, Eisner MP, Kosary CL, Hankey BF, Miller BA, Clegg L, Mariotto A, Feuer EJ, Edwards BK (eds). SEER Cancer Statistics Review, 1975-2002, National Cancer Institute. Bethesda, MD

Now, in general, RCC is typically diagnosed in the seventh decade of life, with a median age at diagnosis of 65 (which is a statistical way of saying that about half the people diagnosed with RCC are older than 65 and half are younger than 65). If we look at the figure provided, we quickly notice that RCC is extremely rare before the age of 35 and the rates increase sharply thereafter. Looking even closer, we notice that RCC incidence rates peak around the age 75 and then drop off slightly in the ninth decade of life. The take home message here is that the development of RCC is a much more common occurrence as the population ages. Not exactly an earth shattering observation, but interesting nonetheless, especially given that more people these days are living well into their late sixties, seventies and eighties. Now if you want to test your reasoning skills, see if you can postulate as to why the rates fall as people enter their nineties. Is there something about being ninety that protects a person from RCC or do you think it's some other, less biological, explanation? I won't tell you the answer but I'll give you a hint...my money is on the latter explanation.

While the increasing incidence rates with increasing age don't set off any trumpets or fanfares, something that does raise eyebrows and draw attention to RCC is what has happened to these incidence rates over time. According to data from the National Cancer Institute, the overall incidence rate of RCC in the U.S. has increased steadily each year since the early 1970's (Reis, 2005). Early on, some people argued that perhaps this trend was simply due to the fact that screening technologies have become very advanced and we are just a whole lot better at finding RCCs than we used to be. While this idea does probably explain some of the increase, there have been some very elegant studies that have shown that this explanation cannot account for all of the increase that we have seen over the past three decades (Chow, 1999). In other words, there is strong evidence that RCC incidence rates are truly on the rise because more people are actually developing the disease and not just that we are better at finding and diagnosing them. More recently there have been some rumblings that these rates are actually beginning to fall, but it is simply too early to tell if this is true and the general consensus is that RCC is a cancer for which incidence rates are on the rise.

What's even more interesting than the overall increase in incidence over time is what we see if we look at these increasing trends across categories of gender and race. Figure 2 charts the increasing incidence rates for RCC individually for white males (•—•), black males (♦—♦), white females (■—■) and black females (▲—▲). The first thing that jumps right out is that the incidence rates appear to be steadily rising for all four groups.

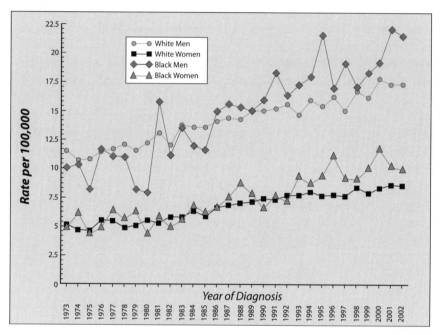

FIGURE 2:   Incidence Rates for RCC Across Gender and Racial Groups
This graph shows the incidence rates for white men (●—●), white women (■—■), black men (◆—◆) and black women (▲—▲). Of particular note is the steady increasing trend in RCC incidence across all four groups over the past thirty years. In addition, notice how the rates for blacks have eventually surpassed that of whites over the last decade.

Ries LAG, Eisner MP, Kosary CL, Hankey BF, Miller BA, Clegg L, Mariotto A, Feuer EJ, Edwards BK (eds). SEER Cancer Statistics Review, 1975-2002, National Cancer Institute. Bethesda, MD

    Upon closer inspection though, there is something else we can glean from this simple figure. Among both men and women, incidence rates for blacks have in more recent years surpassed that of whites. This simple observation gives rise to a myriad of questions: is this explained by the fact that over the past three decades blacks have achieved better access to health care and therefore a better chance of being diagnosed with RCC? Maybe some risk factor for the development of RCC has become more prevalent in blacks than whites in recent decades? While looking at data like those presented in the above figure cannot answer these questions, they do provide the initial inquiry that leads to more focused and sophisticated investigations that can help to answer these questions. My point here is that simply by looking at standard descriptive statistics, not only can we better gauge the true impact of RCC but we can also generate important questions that will ultimately lead to a better understanding of this troublesome cancer.

RCC MORTALITY

Any discussion of the public health impact of a cancer (or any disease for that matter) would be remiss if it did not include a discussion of *mortality rates*. While incidence rates focus on the number of new cancers diagnosed in a given population for a given time period, mortality rates focus on the number of people actually dying from that cancer in the same population over the same time period. Indeed, there are many people that argue that mortality rates are a better measure of the burden of a cancer in a particular population. After all, being diagnosed with cancer is only half the equation. There is the issue of how lethal a cancer is once it is diagnosed. As such, mortality rates are often used in combination with incidence rates to give additional insight into how effective we are at treating a particular cancer. For instance, incidence rates of pancreatic cancer are similar to that of oral cancer (about 11 cases per 100,000), so one might conclude that these two cancers have an equal impact on society. A comparison of mortality rates though reveals that the mortality rate for pancreatic cancer (11 deaths per 100,000) is nearly four times that of oral cancer (3 deaths per 100,000), thereby unmasking pancreatic cancer as the more deadly malignancy. Before we start championing mortality rates as the better means of measuring the impact of cancer, we should mention that they have their limitations too. Mortality rates rely heavily on our ability to get accurate data on causes of death. Even in a patient with a known cancer diagnosis it is often not straightforward as to whether the cancer was irrelevant, an underlying cause or a contributing cause to the patient's death. The other limitation is that mortality rates do not provide information on the number of people living with cancer, which is undoubtedly a burden on both the individual and society. In essence, the reality of the situation is that which statistic (incidence or mortality) is more revealing is a matter of personal opinion. Regardless of which side of the fence you come down on, there is no denying that both incidence and mortality rates (especially when used together) provide an informative window for viewing the impact of cancer.

Turning back to our friends at the American Cancer Society, we find that they expect about 14,000 deaths this year in the U.S. that will be attributed to RCC. The overall mortality rate for RCC in the U.S. is about 4 deaths per 100,000 individuals (for reference, compare that with prostate cancer at 11 deaths per 100,000 and breast cancer at 15 deaths per 100,000) (Reis, 2005). Now recall earlier when we compared incidence rates and saw that the rates for prostate and breast were about six times higher than RCC. Well, the story has changed a bit now that we look at mortality rates hasn't it? When we compare mortality rates (which remember, some people argue are better measures of the impact of a disease) we see that the rates for breast and prostate are only about three times higher than that of RCC. Couple that with the fact that RCC mortality rates appear to be holding steady or rising slightly while mortality rates for breast and prostate are falling, and now we aren't so inclined to discredit the impact of RCC in relation to these bigger, certainly more publicized, cancers. So why did the story change so much when we move from incidence to mortality rates? Basically, it can be attributed in part to the fact that screening for breast and prostate cancer is very successful (i.e. we find these tumors early when they are more treatable) and there are a lot of very effective treatments out there for these cancers. In contrast, there is no screening method for RCC (i.e. a considerable portion are found at an advanced stage) and unfortunately there are currently only limited treatment options for RCC patients. Essentially, RCC is a classic example of why we need to withhold judgment about the impact of a cancer until all the votes are in, so to speak.

OTHER MEASURES OF THE IMPACT OF RCC
The complexity in assessing the true impact of a cancer by simply looking at incidence and mortality rates illustrated in the previous two sections has generated some interest in developing other, perhaps more accurate ways to measure cancer burden (Burnett, 2005). Concepts such as "years of life lost" try to factor in the fundamental difference between cancers that affect younger populations (e.g. leukemia) and those that primarily affect older populations (e.g. prostate cancer). Basically, these statistics are generated by comparing survival times from people with a particular cancer to the life expectancy of a similar individual using actuarial tables. For RCC, it is estimated that the average number of years of life lost for RCC patients is about 12.8 years. That is to say, RCC on average takes away about 12.8 years from those people diagnosed with the disease. Compare that with 20.1 years for brain cancer, 13.5 years for breast cancer, 11.8 years for lung cancer,

9.8 years for colon cancer and 6.1 years for prostate cancer (Burnett, 2005). To go even further, some researchers have championed the use of measures like "disability-adjusted life years" that try to not only assess the impact of a cancer based on years lost to death but also on the quality of life for those that have to live with the disease. So by now it should be pretty clear that putting a final label on how important a cancer is in a particular population is not exactly a straightforward process and can be dependent on how one looks at the numbers.

At this point you may be asking what is the take home message with regard to the impact of RCC? First of all, it bears repeating that we should always withhold judgment on the impact a cancer, or any disease, has on a population until we've really looked closely at the statistics and made some important comparisons. Also, we have to remember that there are many ways to measure "disease burden" and which measure is more telling is a matter of personal opinion. Having said that, it's clear that, from an epidemiological standpoint, RCC is a cancer with some very unique and distinguishing characteristics. Perhaps most notably, RCC represents a cancer for which incidence and mortality rates have been rising at a steady rate for more than three decades. Layer on top of that the notion that RCC typically strikes people in their early to mid 60s and the overall burden of this cancer grows more pronounced. It is these very characteristics that have helped to place RCC into a small handful of cancers that are currently on the National Cancer Institute's "watch list" for the next decade. As such, there is a great deal of attention being given to addressing important issues related to the entire natural history of RCC, from how to better diagnose and treat this malignancy to issues of quality of life once treatment has been initiated. Specific to this chapter however, there is currently a particular emphasis being placed on improving our understanding of why and how RCC develops. Explicitly, we need to better understand what puts a person at risk of developing RCC. What things do people do (or not do) on a regular basis that might serve to increase the chances that they will develop RCC? By improving our knowledge of what factors are associated with an increased risk of developing RCC, we have the potential not only to learn more about the inner-workings of this cancer but also to educate ourselves and others as to how to prevent RCC from ever developing in the first place. As someone once said, sometimes the best offense is a good defense. The remainder of this chapter will focus on the current state of knowledge regarding what environmental and lifestyle factors are associated with an increased risk of developing RCC.

RISK FACTORS FOR RCC

A physician and an epidemiologist are sitting by a riverbank engaged in a conversation. Suddenly, their exchange is disrupted when they notice that the river in front of them is now filling up with thousands of people calling out for help. The physician quickly begins charging towards the water in an effort to pull the drowning victims to safety on the shore. As he runs toward the water he notices that the epidemiologist is not by his side. He turns to find his friend and shouts out to him "Hey, where are you going?" The epidemiologist turns back and yells out, "I'm going up stream to figure out why people are falling in the river in the first place".

The above story is obviously meant for illustrative purposes only. The point being that there are different ways to try to reduce the impact of a particular disease (in our case RCC) on a population. One way is to improve our ability to diagnose and treat it. This no doubt is the primary day-to-day focus of the medical and basic science communities. Another way to reduce disease burden is to figure out why the disease occurs in the first place and try to stop it before it even starts. This approach is often categorized as "prevention and control" and it falls primarily under the purview of epidemiologists and other public health researchers. Now to be sure, which one of these methods is more effective at reducing disease burden will probably depend on whom you are asking. To me, the most logical assessment is that each approach is of equal merit and that our only hope of ever reducing the burden of RCC is to implement both strategies. In this section of the chapter, I am going to try to relay what we currently know about the things that put us at risk of developing RCC and thereby hopefully provide education on ways to reduce this risk. But first, a brief comment about "causes" of disease.

As the cartoon at the start of this chapter alluded to, identifying causes of a disease is a tricky business. Even the philosophical concept of what the word "cause" means has been the subject of entire textbooks (much to my chagrin in graduate school). Let's just say that we need to view everything in the world of science and medicine with the right amount of skepticism. Any physician or researcher who speaks to you in absolutes should be viewed with extreme caution because we all know that the world we live in does not usually deal in black and white. Given that, the one suggestion I would provide in helping you evaluate the level of evidence regarding a proposed cause (or better termed, a 'risk factor') for any disease is that of *validation*. What I mean specifically is that no single study or report is ever enough to claim certainty regarding causation, no matter how many famous names appear on the paper or how reputable the institution may be. We need to see that the results have been validated (i.e. reproduced) over and over again by both the original investigators and, more importantly, other independent investigators. Unfortunately, sometimes the research community gets a bit caught up in focusing on egos rather than ferreting out the truth. This leads to investigators sometimes working against each other, rather than with each other against the disease…but that is a subject for another day. To help us leap off into our discussion of what things put us at risk of developing RCC, we just needed a healthy reminder that there are few things that are certain in this life (I seem to remember something about death and taxes being the only ones). The search for causes of RCC is no different; certainties are indeed rare.

GENETIC SUSCEPTIBILITY TO RCC

Despite what may be the broad public perception, the causes of cancer (and RCC specifically) are primarily related to lifestyle, dietary and environmental exposures and not the inheritance of a gene from one's parents. What I mean by this is that the vast majority of cancers (and RCCs for that matter) are *sporadic* and not *heritable* (i.e. they do not appear to be caused by a sinister gene being passed surreptitiously from parent to child). The studies that have supported this notion are too involved and far beyond the scope of this chapter but suffice to say they consistently point to lifestyle, dietary and other environmental exposures rather than simple family genetics as the cause of most of the cancers in the U.S. Having said that, I do need to clarify two issues. First of all, there are some cases of rare genetic disorders like von Hippel-Lindau syndrome or Birt Hogg Dube' syndrome where it does appear that a single gene is passed from parent to child that dramatically increases the child's risk of developing RCC sometime in their life (Linehan, 2004). These cases however make up an extremely small portion of the RCCs diagnosed in the U.S. each year. The second point is that the notion that most RCCs are not heritable is not to say that genetics is not important in determining who develops RCC. In truth, a person's genetic make-up can be very important in some cases. For instance, we will see in a bit that smoking is a major risk factor for developing RCC. But there are lots of heavy smokers who never develop RCC. What gives? Well, this is where a person's genetics can come into play. Say for example a person carries a particular version of a gene (genes can have many versions called *alleles*) that produces a protein enzyme that is extremely effective at breaking down toxins from cigarette smoke and removing them from the body. Compared to someone without that particular version of the gene, the person carrying the "better version" would be less susceptible to the RCC-causing effects of smoking. So the genes you inherit from your parents can be important in dictating your overall risk of developing RCC. In fact, there have been some targeted efforts to determine how the combination of genes and environment work together to determine a person's risk of developing RCC (Semeza, 2001; Sweeny, 2000). The take home point, however, is that the concept that RCC (and cancer in general) is primarily caused by a single, nefarious gene being passed silently from generation to generation is very rarely the case. For that reason, I often take issue when the media reports that researchers have found a new "cancer gene". The purpose of a gene is not to cause cancer. Each gene is designed to produce a protein that will carry out a specific job that we need to live on this earth. Cancer arises when we lose control of these genes through a mutation or some other phenomenon that alters the way the protein that gene makes is supposed to work. So given that, the germane question for us becomes what causes these alterations deep within the cells of the kidney that ultimately makes them go out of control? For part of the answer, we need only look as far as the world around us.

MAJOR RISK FACTORS FOR RCC

With the role of genetics in somewhat better perspective, this is where the rubber finally hits the road and we get to find out what it is that you and I do on a daily basis that might increase our risk of developing RCC. First though (I heard that collective groan...just bear with me), we should mention exactly how it is that these risk factors for RCC are identified as such. In general, there are two primary study designs that epidemiologists use to help determine the relationship between a putative risk factor and a disease (in our case, RCC). The first type of investigation is called a *case-control* study. In these investigations we identify a group of people with RCC (the cases) and a comparable group of people without RCC (the controls). Then we find out information from each of them about the things they are exposed to in their everyday lives (i.e. what do they eat, do they smoke, do they exercise, what was their weight at different ages in their lives, etc.). Obviously, I'm oversimplifying the process but you get the idea. We can then compare the data between the two groups and see if there are any really interesting differences between what one group reports versus what the other group reports (again, in the interest of time,

I'm really oversimplifying a very involved statistical process). One concern with this design is that the cases, because of the impact of their cancer diagnosis, might be motivated to do a better job of recalling their exposures and lifestyle choices than the controls individuals who remain cancer free. Given this caveat, we try to do everything we can to make sure each group is reporting the information as accurately as possible. At the end of the day, we must always remember that this is a limitation of case-control studies. For this reason, the case-control design is often considered to be slightly weaker at establishing a causal relationship compared to the other major epidemiologic study design, the *cohort* study. In a cohort study, we organize a large group of cancer-free individuals (usually numbering in the tens of thousands), get them to tell us about the things they are exposed to in their everyday lives and then follow-up them up over several years to determine who develops RCC and who doesn't. The strength here is that everyone is cancer free at the start so we don't have to worry about people recalling exposures differently. For this reason, the cohort design is considered a much more scientifically sound design compared to the case-control study. One major drawback however is that cohort studies take a lot more time to complete compared to case-control studies, mainly because in cohort studies we have to wait for people to develop RCC. The other drawback is that because RCC is a relatively rare occurrence, the cohort studies require larger amounts of people to enroll in the study and this translates to a larger overall cost of the study. All in all, both study designs have played an important role over the past three decades in helping to establish the risk factors for developing RCC. So, finally, let's take a look at what we know about risk factors for RCC.

Obesity
    Probably the most consistent finding with regard to RCC risk factors is the notion that obesity (typically defined by a body mass index of > 30 kg/m^2)[ii] increases a person's risk of developing RCC (reviewed in Linbald and Adami, 2002). Early on, there was some speculation that the risk might actually be stronger for women than men. Over the past five years though, the consensus has become that the increase in risk is pretty much the same for both men and women. Essentially, those individuals who have a history of obesity are at about two to three times the risk of developing RCC as people in the "normal" body mass index range (18-24 kg/m^2). Now, remember how we said that validation was important in establishing something as a cause of RCC? Well, to date there are about

40 studies (mostly case-control but there are several cohort investigations too) that have shown an increase in risk of RCC for obese individuals. In 2004, the largest cohort study to date on this issue was published (Bjorge, 2004). The study was conducted in Norway and involved follow-up of over two million men and women. The authors concluded that the risk of RCC increased with increasing body mass index level for both genders. This study coupled with the large number of previous studies, firmly establishes that obesity increases a person's risk of developing RCC. So what now? First of all, we'd like to know exactly how obesity increases the risk of RCC since it's pretty clear that it does. Therefore, we are now designing studies that will help us peer inside the body and figure out how something like obesity works within the body (and the kidney cells in particular) to cause RCC. In addition, there are some interesting studies that are beginning to look closely at whether weight change over a lifetime is important. Similarly, some investigators are looking at the question of whether being obese during certain periods of your life (e.g. adolescence vs. adulthood) is more dangerous than others with regard to the risk of developing RCC. From a public health standpoint we also need to know whether losing weight reduces the risk back down to that of a non-obese person. So while obesity may be the most established risk factor for RCC, clearly there is still a lot of work to be done to ferret out some interesting nuances of this well-known association.

SMOKING

Now I know you're not gonna believe this but hold onto your hats...smoking is bad for you. I know, shocking isn't it? All sarcasm aside, the only other widely established risk factor for RCC is that good old public health scourge itself, cigarette smoking. Now what might actually surprise you is that the concept that smoking causes all types of cancer is not exactly correct. In fact there are only a handful of cancers for which smoking is considered an established risk factor; and RCC is one of them. How established one might ask? Well in their recent report entitled *The Health Consequences of Smoking*, the Department of Health and Human Services confirmed that there is now sufficient evidence to declare a causal relationship between smoking and the development of RCC (http://www.dhhs.gov). Indeed, the authors of the report acknowledged that "smoking is an established cause of RCC and a substantial number of cases could be avoided through smoking prevention and cessation". Of interest, this same sentiment was echoed in an earlier international report released in 2004 by the International

Agency for Research on Cancer that characterized the evidence of a causal association between smoking and RCC as wholly sufficient (IARC, 2004). Moreover, authors of a recent study that looked at data from 26 epidemiological investigations spanning 35 years concluded that "inhaled tobacco smoke is undoubtedly implicated in the etiology (the development) of RCC, with a strong dose dependent increase in risk associated with number of cigarettes smoked per day" (Hunt, 2005). Clearly, there is no question that RCC is now firmly established in the scientific and medical community as a smoking-related disease.

As is the case with obesity, there remain several important and pressing questions regarding the nature and inner-workings of how smoking increases the risk of RCC that need to be addressed. Interestingly, it appears that once a person quits smoking their risk of RCC drops steadily. In fact, after about 15 years from the point of smoking cessation, the overall risk appears to be back to that of a never smoker (Parker, 2003). Other issues to be addressed over the next decade include (1) what are the molecular changes that occur within the kidney cells of smokers that lead to RCC and (2) are there any subgroups within smokers where the risk is especially high (e.g. overweight smokers)? By focusing intense efforts on these important issues, researchers hope to provide the opportunity to broaden our understanding of smoking-related RCC and ultimately use this knowledge to impact on the prevention and treatment of RCC.

HYPERTENSION

While the message regarding the risk of RCC associated with obesity and smoking is very straightforward, the story with hypertension (high blood pressure) is a bit more complicated. Often referred to as "the other risk factor for RCC", a history of hypertension does appear to increase the risk of RCC by about 30-50%. What makes it so complicated however is that there is a long-standing debate regarding whether it is hypertension or the medications used to treat hypertension that is the cause of this increase in risk. To cut right to the point, it appears now that there is a very strong argument that it is actually hypertension itself that increases the risk of RCC. To help lay this controversy to rest, some very astute researchers designed studies to directly address this issue (Yuan, 1998; Chow, 2000; Yu and Ross, 2001; Fryzek, 2005). Basically, they looked at groups of individuals who had never taken any antihypertensive medication. Within this specific group they found that compared to people with no history of hypertension, those with hypertension were indeed at increased risk of RCC. Then they flipped things around and looked at people that took antihypertensive medications for conditions other than high blood pressure and found no evidence that these medications increased the risk of RCC. Pretty convincing evidence that hypertension is the real culprit. Regardless, the debate does rage on in some circles. However, what just about everyone does agree on is that people with a history of hypertension (whether it is because of the hypertension or the medication used to treat it) are at increased risk of developing RCC.

THE BIG THREE

At this point, if you walk away from this chapter with nothing else, at least you should know that smoking, obesity and hypertension are considered three main risk factors for RCC. Cut these out of your daily lives and your risk of RCC decreases sharply. To add some perspective to this, there were some elegant studies conducted in the mid to late 1990's to get an idea of exactly how important these risk factors are in the development of RCC from a public health standpoint (McLaughlin, 1995; Yu, 1998; Benichou, 1998). From those studies, the general consensus was that these three factors combined to account for about 50% of the RCCs that are diagnosed in the U.S. every year. Put another way, if we could eliminate smoking, obesity and hypertension then the number of RCCs we see in the U.S. would be cut in half. Now of course, we are not going to be able to do that any time in the near future (maybe never), so I mentioned it more as a means of driving home the point that these three factors are major players in determining a person's risk of developing RCC. Which obviously begs the question, if these three account for 50% of the RCCs...what accounts for the other 50%?

EMERGING RISK FACTORS FOR RCC

I wish there was more to tell in this section but unfortunately this is currently an area of research that is, shall we say, in progress. Remember that we said in order to firmly establish a particular factor as a true cause of (or risk factor for) a disease, one of the most important things we look for is validation over a large number of studies. Well, there are a lot of researchers working towards amassing the kind of data that will be required to help ferret out other causes (or protective factors for that matter) of RCC. There are however, a few candidates that based on some early returns are looking pretty interesting. Before we jump into those, let's quickly mention a couple of things have been looked at pretty extensively and been found to NOT increase the risk of RCC. Neither coffee nor tea consumption has been convincingly associated with the risk of developing RCC (reviewed in Linbald and Adami, 2002). Similarly, it doesn't look like artificial sweeteners affect the risk of RCC either (reviewed in Linbald and Adami, 2002). With those out of the way, so to speak, we can move on to looking a bit closer at those interesting candidates I mentioned above.

ALCOHOL

While early investigators suggested that alcohol might increase the risk of RCC, studies over the past 5-10 years have actually shown a fairly consistent inverse association, meaning that as alcohol consumption goes up, the risk of RCC goes down (Wolk, 1996; Parker 2002; Nicodemus, 2004; Mahabir, 2005). Of course, we have to be very careful with this public health message but it does appear, as with cardiovascular disease, that a few drinks a week may actually protect your kidney from RCC. So nowadays, I tell my friends and family that all those late night sojourns to the pubs in college were just an attempt to protect my kidney. In all seriousness, we will need to wait and see what the story is five to ten years from now when more studies have weighed in on the issue. If it can be firmly established that moderate alcohol consumption does protect from RCC, this information could be used in public health intervention efforts among high-risk populations. What's more, it might give clues to help guide the next wave of efforts to develop drugs to prevent and treat RCC.

URINARY TRACT INFECTIONS

A history of urinary tract infections (UTIs) is an accepted risk factor for bladder cancer and some early studies are suggesting that this may also be the case for RCC (Murai, 2004). Our own data have even suggested that this risk may be much more pronounced in men and smokers (Parker, 2004). One hypothesis to explain this association is that the bacteria that are known to cause the vast majority of UTIs (*E. coli*) produce a substance that causes cells to make an excess of a particular protein (called cyclooxygenase-2) that is particularly favorable to cancer progression. One problem is that the studies so far linking UTIs to RCC have all been case-control studies and there is some concern that patients with RCC are more likely to recall having a UTI than their non-cancer counterparts. Therefore, we will need to wait until more studies, particularly cohort studies, can provide data to better establish the role that urinary tract infections play in RCC development.

PHYSICAL ACTIVITY

There have been a couple of recent studies that have shown a link between physical activity and a reduced risk of RCC (Menenez, 2004; van Dijk, 2004; Mahabir, 2004; Nicodemus, 2004). Unfortunately, we have to be mindful that some earlier studies reported no such association (Bergstrom, 2001; Mellemgaard, 1995). What makes this particular risk factor a bit more difficult to study is that physical activity is very highly correlated with other risk factors for RCC, namely obesity and smoking. Therefore it is often difficult to conclude whether the association (or lack of an association in some studies) might be due to the close relationship of physical activity with these other factors. There are more data on the way as several investigators have designed studies to look at this question. My take on the current skepticism regarding this issue is that we all know physical activity is something we should be doing for our overall health anyway and if it also reduces the risk of RCC, well then all the more reason to get out there and get exercising.

DIET

Citing the well-reported differences in RCC incidence rates between Western and Asian countries (see the discussion of incidence rates earlier in this chapter), the hypothesis was raised quite a while ago that diet could play a role in RCC development given that one of the distinguishing features of these two regions (besides ethnicity of course) is the foods that are typically consumed. In spite of some inconsistencies and controversial findings that have been reported over the last two decades, there is a considerable amount of data to suggest that a diet high in vegetable and fruit consumption reduces the risk of developing RCC (reviewed in Linbald and Adami, 2002). A large number of specific foods and nutrients have been analyzed for their association with RCC but, to date, there has been nothing that has reached the consistency of the data supporting fruits and vegetables. As one can imagine, diet is very difficult to study because it requires people to recall what they have eaten over long periods of time (and I sometimes have a hard time remembering what I ate for breakfast). Regardless, the methods for improving recall of dietary consumption among study participants are getting better and the general feeling is that as more studies are conducted we will be able to get a better handle on what other food items might play a role in altering one's risk of developing RCC.

REPRODUCTIVE AND HORMONAL FACTORS

There is some evidence that certain hormone-related factors may affect a woman's risk of developing RCC. The use of oral contraceptives and estrogen replacement has been linked, albeit weakly, to an increased risk of RCC (reviewed in Linbald and Adami, 2002). Interestingly, there is some growing data to suggest that reproductive factors such as age at menarche, number of births and age at menopause are all associated with RCC risk. One unifying theory that could help to tie these all together is that the longer a woman is exposed to estrogen, the greater her risk of RCC. The theory is based on data suggesting that as the body metabolizes estrogen and excretes the remains, the waste by-products can be harmful to genes in certain tissues. This is often referred to as the "estrogen metabolism hypothesis" in other cancers affecting women only (McPherson, 1996). In fact, some investigators are currently trying to assess whether those women who are better at removing these estrogen waste products might be at lower risk of RCC compared to women who do not remove these byproducts quickly and efficiently. It bears re-emphasizing that this is only a hypothesis and as such needs to be tested rigorously before any decision about its veracity can be made. However, it is becoming clearer that certain hormone-related factors appear to be associated with the risk of RCC.

RARE OCCUPATIONAL EXPOSURES

Finally, we should briefly mention that there are a few rare exposures that have also been associated with an increased risk of RCC. Most of these are very specific occupational exposures and therefore are not going to affect the vast majority of readers of this book. Interestingly, RCC is not widely considered an "occupational cancer" since most of the studies that have focused on certain groups of workers rarely report an elevated number of RCCs in these populations. Regardless, some of these specific factors should be quickly mentioned, as there are some data that suggest a role for them in the development of RCC. Moore et al (2005) provide an excellent review of the current state of knowledge regarding these types of exposures and RCC. An elevated risk of RCC has been reported for workers exposed to asbestos and interestingly enough, asbestos fibers can cause RCC in laboratory animals. Several studies have also reported an increased risk for exposure to gasoline and other petroleum products however there are studies that show no association as well. Other rare exposures that may increase the risk of RCC include certain solvents (especially chlorinated ones), diesel exhaust, polycyclic hydrocarbons, printing dyes, cadmium and lead. In truth, the list of these items that have been associated with RCC is quite long (Moore, 2005) however the data for most is scant at best, often not validated and ultimately of less consequence due to the rare nature of these exposures. In essence, for most of us these are not the exposures we need to worry about.

SUMMARY

On the whole, fewer and fewer people seem to give much thought to cancer prevention. In turn, most want to focus on developing better, more effective treatments for cancer. In truth, I myself have become increasingly more interested in performing experiments in the lab and running clinical trials rather than conducting classic epidemiologic studies of RCC. Recently, a longtime friend and mentor of mine was listening to me rave on and on about the vast potential of some new therapeutic approach that I was sure would eventually lead to the development of amazing new possibilities for treating RCC patients. In his usual accommodating manner, he let me finish my thoughts and quickly validated my enthusiasm for the potential to harness this method in order to reduce the burden of RCC. Then he subtly reminded me of another effective approach to reducing the impact of RCC. He said, "So, now tell me, what are you doing to better understand why RCC occurs in the first place?"

In this chapter I have attempted to provide you, the reader, with a brief introduction to the epidemiology (i.e. the *where, when* and *why*) of RCC. The reality is that an entire book could be dedicated to this subject, so there is only so much that can be accomplished in one single chapter. Hopefully, the overall message that comes through is that while RCC is a relatively rare cancer, it is one that undeniably has an impact on our society. Perhaps more to the point, the impact of this cancer appears to be rising steadily. This clearly underscores the need to focus efforts on reducing the burden of RCC by flushing out the various risk factors for the disease. To date, we know a good deal about what things put us at risk of developing RCC, but there is much more work to be done. Researchers over the next few decades will need to concentrate on identifying new risk factors for RCC as well as improving our understanding of how the known risk factors work within the cells of the kidney to ultimately cause cancer. That way we would have the potential to stop this cancer by never letting it start.

i   Incidence rates are usually reported as "age-adjusted incidence rates" so that they can be compared across different populations that many have very different age make-ups. For instance, we would not want to directly compare incidence rates between Boca Raton, Florida (where the population has a large percentage of people in their 70's and 80's) and Chapel Hill, North Carolina (a college town where the population is decidedly more on the spring chicken side) without accounting for the difference in age make-up.

ii   Body mass index is calculated by dividing a person's weight in kilograms by their height in meters squared. The basic idea is that this gives a better indication (although certainly not perfect) of body fat composition than does just a regular weight.

NOTES:

NOTES:

CHAPTER 8
Our Journey *with* Kidney Cancer
by Pat *and* Gene Upshaw

This is *Pat.*

In February, 2001, I went in for my yearly check up. I had been tired and just not feeling well. I thought the reason was my grief over losing my mother who had passed away in January. I had also lost a few pounds. The doctor ordered blood work that showed I was anemic. He then ordered a colonoscopy that showed nothing. My blood levels continued to get lower so he put me on a higher dose of iron. But, by June, I was clearly getting worse. I was more tired and had no color. I went back to the doctor and told him that I was sick. He did more blood work and a urine test, got the results, and told me there was nothing new.

In July, we went to the lake. The temperature outside was over 100 degrees but I was cold and couldn't get warm. Gene wrapped me in a blanket and made a fire but I just couldn't get warm. The next week, at work, I noticed a bump on my arm and thought that a mosquito had bitten me. Then the bump turned into a rash that spread over both of my arms and my back. I went to the doctor again and reported all of this. He put me on steroids for a week. That didn't help. I was using calamine lotion and benadryl to try to control the rash. Then, I started getting night sweats even though I never sweat, not even in hot weather. My night clothes would be wet from drenching sweat.

So, I went back to the doctor again on July 9, 2001, and told him that I knew something was wrong. He said he would do a blood test to rule out lupus and cancer but that he didn't think that it was cancer. He also ordered a CT scan for 1 p.m. that day. At 3:30 that afternoon, the doctor called and said that he needed to see me for follow up. A spot had shown up on the CT scan.

On Friday, July 13, my family and I went to the doctor. It turned out that the spot was a five inch tumor on my left kidney. The doctor had already made an appointment for me to see an oncologist and a surgeon on the following Tuesday, July 17. My daughter asked me to change the appointment to a different surgeon whom she knew so I did.

On Tuesday, July 17, we went to see the oncologist at 9 a.m. After testing a sample of my blood, he told me that I needed three pints of blood that day. We left there and went to my 10:30 appointment with the surgeon. He showed us the size of the tumor and told us what he would do. We left there and went to the hospital for the three pints of blood.

On Thursday, July 19, at 3 p.m., I went into surgery. Afterwards, the doctor told my family that the surgery had gone as well as could be expected and that he had been able to remove about 96 to 97% of the cancer. I was in ICU for three days then transferred to a standard hospital room. I could not stand to smell food or to drink water. I just wanted to go home. Finally, I was discharged from the hospital but, at home, I still could not eat or drink water. I was hurting and felt very sick. After four days, Gene said I had to go back to the hospital so they could figure out what was going on. I didn't know anything about what was happening.

This is *Gene.*

We took her back into the hospital. She really didn't know anything about what was going on. Pat was really out of it so I took her to the emergency room. They put her back in a room and started out by administering morphine to give her some relief from the pain. She was in serious pain and pretty bad condition. They kept her in the hospital and, after about three days there, she was still so sedated by the drugs that she didn't know anything. I was really at my wit's end. They had her so drugged that she didn't know what she was doing. Friends and family would stay with her during the day so that I could get some work done in my small business. I would go up every evening at about five o'clock and spend the night on a small bed in the room with her so that I could keep an eye on her. It was a disaster. Pat didn't know what she was doing. She'd wake up every thirty to sixty minutes and I would catch her trying to climb the wall because she didn't know where she was. After a couple of days, it became evident that she was badly dehydrated so they put a pit line in. That was a horrible experience. It took four or five of us to hold her down. As a matter of fact, it got so bad that I had to leave the room. It was a bloody mess but they finally inserted the pit line and started administering more drugs including morphine. By the third day, they had to put a little tube down her nose to feed her. Four more days went by and her eyes started closing involuntarily. She was sent down for a brain scan because they thought possibly she might have a tumor on the brain.

Tumor on the brain. Boy, was I a basket case then. But, I think what it all boiled down to was the morphine she was on. One of the nurses told me she needed to get off the morphine and start learning how to deal with the pain. Within a day or so, the morphine was shut off. I worked with her every night and stayed till about nine every morning. That way, I had a chance to see all of the doctors and to visit with them. I finally told them that we needed to get Pat fixed up, she was on the downhill road. For the next few days they worked with her, discontinuing the medications. So, with a little bit of work and the grace of God, we worked through it and got her off the morphine and the other drugs. After about ten to twelve days in the hospital, I finally got to bring her home.

In the hospital, Pat had been given a protein drink that she didn't mind too much. So, I found out from the hospital how to get it since it wasn't available in Wichita. I had to order it from California so I ordered a case. As far as I'm concerned, the drink really helped her and probably kept her alive. It was about the only thing she could drink or even would drink. She convalesced for about thirteen or fourteen weeks then was able to go back to work.

When Pat came home from the hospital the second time, a couple of months went by and then, sometime in November or December, she started to have quite a bit of pain very high up in her chest. The pain was so severe she could hardly lie down at night. The doctor suspected gall bladder problems so he ran her through the gall bladder tests but couldn't find anything. Then he suspected liver cancer and put her through some more tests but couldn't find anything. The testing went on for two or three weeks off and on while the pain really messed up her eating and sleeping habits. The pain was so severe she'd cry if she tried to lie down. She took a lot of antacids trying to get relief but they didn't help. The doctors couldn't figure out what was causing the pain. Finally, the pain subsided on its own.

Shortly after that, we started investigating and using herbs and whatnot. Pat has used the herbs regularly since then. It's been a few years now and the pain's not come back. We still don't understand what happened and neither do the doctors. But, it's gone. We don't know if the herbs are helping but we know they're not hurting and Pat feels better. So, we'll keep on doing what we're doing and thank the good Lord for Pat's health.

After we started her on some herbs, I began to check out natural remedies. Pat started taking a lot of vitamins and we set up more herbs for her to start taking. We've been working with this and she's held her own for about four years. I'm not proud of the blood tests but the doctors don't seem too concerned. Everything's okay as far as they're concerned.

Still, after three years, she's kept slowly going downhill. So, now I've started her on essential oils that she rubs into her feet. There're three different kinds made by a company I'm not going to name here but if anybody would like to talk to me, they can always call me and I'll talk with them about it. We've been doing that for about six or eight months. We don't know if it's helping or not but she's still holding her own on blood tests. The last time couple of times that we went back to see the doctor, he was pretty tickled about the blood tests. I still didn't see any kind of improvement in her blood work but her vital signs are okay and holding their own.

Still trying to keep Pat as strong as we can, a friend and I got into some research on a root and started brewing it. After she was drinking the root tea for about four to five weeks, we went back in for another blood test. She, in the meantime had had a spot between the lung and the chest wall that they didn't tell us about in the radiology report about two years ago because it was too small. But, this time, in 2005, they told us about it. After she had been drinking this tea for about four to five weeks, her blood tests showed quite a bit of improvement and the spot was smaller. Basically, of all the things we've done, this tea is the best hope for improvement that we've found in the last four years. We'll have to wait and see. We have another test coming up in about three months and we'll reevaluate it then.

Anyway, this has been chaos and we wish we were more educated about the medical field. There's a doggone lot to learn. But sometimes, you just need to let the good Lord take his course and you have to use your own judgment and take hold of your own life. That's what we've been doing, just trying to use natural ways to heal Pat's body.

We appreciate the opportunity to tell our story.

NOTES:

NOTES:

CHAPTER 9
Psychosocial Issues *of* Renal Cell Cancer
by Steve Ames, Ph.D.

When Cynthia invited me to write a chapter on the psychosocial issues of renal cell carcinoma, we commiserated on the dearth of information specific to renal cell carcinoma and its psychosocial sequelae. We talked about the possibility of writing about studies done on other cancers and translating that information. But, then we decided it would be more meaningful to share with you information about a new study on which I am embarking that is designed to document the consequences of renal cell carcinoma diagnosis on psychosocial functioning and quality of life. This study has several goals but for our purposes here I will focus on the part of the study that specifically looks at the psychosocial consequences of a diagnosis of renal cell carcinoma.

It has been well documented that diagnosis and treatment of other forms of cancer have significant negative consequences on psychosocial functioning and QOL (quality of life). However, there has been a minimal amount of attention given to investigation of the psychosocial and QOL consequences of RCC. Gathering this information is critical to better understand the treatment needs of this patient population and, if warranted, to develop behavioral interventions designed to address needs that may exist. The long-term health objective of this work is to alleviate psychological distress and improve the QOL of individuals with localized RCC.

This investigation will include a total of 60 adults (> 18 years of age) with localized RCC (i.e, stage 1 or 2 or fully resectable stage 3). Focus groups containing 4-6 participants per group will be conducted to gather information about the psychosocial needs of individuals with RCC. Participants will also be administered self-report measures designed to assess psychological symptoms including anxiety, depressive symptoms, psychological distress, and both general and disease specific quality of life prior to nephrectomy and during a 6-month follow-up period. Repeat assessment will be conducted at 1-, 3-, and 6-month follow-up visits. This investigation will include addressing the following aims:

>Evaluate the psychosocial treatment needs of individuals with localized renal cell carcinoma. Treatment needs will be evaluated using qualitative data derived from focus groups and quantitative data from self-reported measures administered to individuals over a 6-month assessment period.
>
>Determine whether anxiety, depressive symptoms, psychological distress, and general and disease specific quality of life change from pre-nephrectomy over a 6-month post-nephrectomy time period.

It is our thought that post-nephrectomy anxiety, depressive symptoms, and psychological distress will be greater, and general and disease specific quality of life will be lower from pre-nephrectomy levels at every assessment point over the 6-month follow-up time period. This study is designed to prove or disprove this idea.

Prior research with other populations of cancer patients have found diagnosis and treatment of the disease has substantial psychological consequences that impact quality of life (QOL). However, at present the psychosocial needs of individuals with renal cell carcinoma (RCC) are unclear and no prior investigations have been conducted to comprehensively assess the psychosocial needs of these individuals. Developing an understanding of the psychosocial needs of individuals with RCC is critical given that individuals with other forms of cancer have been found to have substantial psychosocial needs. Additionally, investigating the psychosocial needs of individuals with RCC is essential in order to advance our understanding of whether unmet psychosocial needs exist which may have a deleterious impact on the quality of life of this patient population. If unmet needs are found to exist, then more specific information is needed to develop behavioral interventions to enhance the QOL of these individuals.

The impact of renal cell carcinoma (RCC) on psychosocial facets of QOL has been understudied, particularly in comparison to the attention psychological aspects of QOL have been given in other forms of cancer. A review of the published literature yielded a total of 5 studies pertaining to the topic investigating the psychosocial needs or QOL of individuals with RCC. However, it is important to highlight that all of these 5 studies focused exclusively on psychosocial and QOL differences between patients receiving different forms of treatment including a phase 1 trial of a autologous tumor-derived vaccine (Cohen, de Moor, Parker, & Amato, 2002), partial versus radical nephrectomy (Clark, Schover, Uzzo, Hafez, Rybicki, & Novick, 2001; Ficarra et al., 2002), or interleukin-2 and/or interferon-alpha cancer therapy (Capuron, Ravaud, Miller, & Dantzer, 2004; Heinzer, Mir, Hulan, & Hulan, 1999). Since the primary aim of these studies was to either compare the differential impact of treatment or the impact of a specific form of treatment on QOL their findings are of limited utility in understanding the psychosocial needs of RCC patients in general. Nevertheless, despite these limitations, 3 of the 5 studies revealed that treatment of RCC can have a significant negative impact on a variety of aspects of psychosocial functioning and QOL (Heinzer et al., 1999), depressive symptoms (Capuron, et al., 2004), anxiety, mild depression, and social problems (Ficarra et al., 2002). On the other hand, 2 of the 5 studies failed to find significant QOL differences between patients being treated for RCC compared to normative data from age and sex-matched general community samples (Clark, 2001, Cohen et al., 2002).

Our literature review also revealed one randomized clinical trial that applied a behavioral intervention in an effort to enhance the psychological and behavioral adjustment of patients with RCC (de Moor et al., 2002). This study randomly assigned 42 patients with metastatic RCC to an expressive writing or control condition. Participants assigned to the expressive writing group reported significantly less sleep disturbance, better sleep quality and sleep duration, and less daytime dysfunction compared to the control group. However, no statistically significant treatment group differences were found with regard to distress, perceived stress, or mood disturbance. The results of this investigation suggest that behavioral interventions have potential application to enhancing the psychosocial functioning and QOL of individuals with RCC. Given the dearth and methodological limitations of the existing literature that has examined the psychosocial needs and QOL of RCC patients, clearly further exploration of the specific needs of this patient population is warranted.

We anticipate that approximately equal numbers of males and females will be recruited. Focus groups will be conducted to evaluate the psychosocial treatment needs of individuals with RCC. Focus groups will contain 4-6 participants. Every effort will be made to have participants complete a focus group between 4 to 8 weeks post nephrectomy. Recruitment of participants and conduct of focus groups will continue until a total of 60 participants are enrolled. Therefore, the number of focus groups conducted will range between 10-15 groups. Evaluation of psychosocial treatment needs will consist of quantitative data gathered from administration of self-report instruments to focus group participants. Data collected at these focus groups will provide a unique understanding of the experiences and needs of adults with RCC.

The focus group content and methodology is based on recommendations drawn from the focus group methodology literature (Kidd & Parshall, 2000; Krueger & Casey, 2000; Stewart & Shamdasani, 1990). To maximize reliability and validity of the data, focus groups will employ a single, experienced moderator for all groups, all groups will include two members of the research team, detailed notes and audio taping will be made of each session, the same staff member will take notes at all groups, a single individual will content code, and multiple groups will be conducted. Each focus group will contain between 4-6 participants. Participants for these groups will be recruited via being informed of the opportunity to participate in this study from medical staff during return visits. The qualitative aspect of the focus group will last 1 hour and participants will be paid $30 for attending. We estimate an additional 30 minutes will be required for baseline administration of the quantitative self-report measures.

Following completion of the baseline assessment participants will be followed for an additional 6 months. During this follow-up period participants will return for in-person administration of the quantitative self-report measures at 1-, 3-, and 6-month post-baseline visits. Participants who are unable to return for in-person follow-up visits will be sent the self-report measures via mail with a pre-paid return envelope.

Careful thought has gone into structuring the group meetings. This is the format we will be using:

A. Introduction/Ground rules (approximately 5 minutes)
   1. Introduction of moderator.
   2. Moderator reminds group members that the session will last 1 hour.
   3. Moderator explains that during the course of the group each member will be asked to provide both written and verbal feedback.
   4. Moderator explains confidential nature of discussion. Although responses during our discussion will be recorded no information that could identify group members as individuals will be collected. Audio recordings and notes taken will be stored in a secure, locked location. Responses will be recorded only to insure that comments are not missed. Audio and written recordings will be destroyed once the study is complete.
   5. Establishment of ground rules.
      Group members are asked to respect others while they are speaking by not interrupting them. Since everyone's comments are important to us and are being recorded we ask that you speak clearly and talk one at a time.

Group members are asked not to carry on "side conversations".

Group members are asked to respect others' opinions and encourage everyone to participate.

Group members are encouraged to add to a comment that another group member has made if they have had a similar experience or have a different perspective.

Group members are again reminded that everything discussed in the group is confidential. Information others choose to discuss or reveal in the group should not be repeated to others outside the group.

B. Icebreaker (approximately 5 minutes)

1. Group members asked to write their first name on both sides of a folded index card (which will remain in front of them on the table) and introduce themselves.

2. Participants asked to name a famous person they would like to meet and the reason why they want to meet them.

C. Opening Statement (approximately 5 minutes)

1. Appeal for help: "You are the experts on how renal cancer has impacted your life and we believe that we can learn a lot from you. Your experiences and opinions will help us learn more about these issues so that we can develop a treatment program to maximize the quality of your life".

2. Explanation of the purpose of the group: "You might be wondering why we asked you participate in this group and why we are interested in talking to you about your experiences with renal cancer." "We need more information about the way that renal cancer has impacted your life." "To gather information about how treatment of renal cancer has affected you."

D. Topic 1: Renal Cancer (approximately 20 minutes)

1. Participants provided with feedback form that asks them to make a written list of 5 or more ways that they view renal cancer affecting the quality of their life.

2. The following topics will be discussed. The moderator will use follow-up semi-structured prompts to facilitate discussion if needed (e.g., "Please tell me more"; "Could you give me an example?"; "Is there anything else?").

Where do you go for information about renal cancer?

What kind of information is difficult to get?

How has renal cancer affected you? How has renal cancer affected you physically? How has renal cancer affected you psychologically? What have you done to cope with renal cancer? What have members of your support system done to help you?

Think about your experience with renal cancer. In particular, think about factors that have made living with renal cancer easier or more difficult. What has made living with renal cancer easier? What has made living with renal cancer more difficult? What kind of support or help did you need that was difficult to get? What else could your doctors do to help you?

E. Topic 2: Renal Cancer Treatment (approximately 15 minutes)
   1. Participants provided with feedback form that asks them to make a written list of 5 or more ways that they view treatment/surgery for renal cancer affects their quality of their life.
   2. The following topics will be discussed. The moderator will use follow-up semi-structured prompts to facilitate discussion if needed (e.g., "Please tell me more"; "Could you give me an example?"; "Is there anything else?").

   Where do you go for information about treatment options for renal cancer? What kind of information is difficult to get?

   How has surgery for renal cancer affected you? How has surgery for renal cancer affected the quality of your life? What has made undergoing surgery easier for you? What has made surgery more difficult? What kind of support or help did you need that was difficult to get? What additional things could your doctors have done to have helped you? What additional things could your family/friends have done to have helped you?

F. Summary of Discussion (approximately 10 minutes)
   1. Moderator provides a brief oral summary of the discussion from topics 1 and 2.
   Moderator asks group: "Is this an adequate summary?" Summary is then refined based on feedback.
   2. Moderator reviews the purpose of the focus group (i.e., development a better understanding of the psychosocial needs of individuals with renal cancer).
   Moderator asks group: "Have we missed anything?" Follow-up questions asked based on feedback.

G. Closing Comments
1. Moderator informs the group that they are at the end of the time allotted for discussion and asks if there are any questions.
2. Moderator thanks participants for the information they contributed.
    a. Collect written feedback forms. Participants provided with blank envelope and asked to place the two feedback forms inside envelope and seal it. Sealed envelopes are then collected by moderator.
3. Moderator provides payment to participants for attending and for time spent.

Because this study is the first investigation that has sought to understand the psychosocial treatment needs of this group, there is no existing data on the psychological aspects of QOL for this group. Therefore, the results of this study are likely to have a significant impact on the field and, if this patient population is found to have psychosocial needs, will lead to the development of an intervention to enhance the QOL of RCC patients. Alternately, there are also several limitations. Although our methods include a baseline assessment prior to time of surgery, it is not possible to collect a true baseline assessment temporally distant from diagnosis of RCC and removed from the potential psychosocial effects of impending surgery. Thus, the baseline assessment may not be representative of a participant's "true" psychosocial functioning prior to the time of RCC. However, we will compare baseline data to published normative data to evaluate how representative this initial assessment is to that of the general population.

This is a first step in addressing the unmet need to understand the psychosocial treatment needs with the goal of improving the quality of life of RCC patients in general. There is no anticipated immediate benefit for participants volunteering for this protocol. However, the data derived from this study will potentially benefit other patients with RCC in that it may lead to a better understanding of the treatment needs of these individuals and may result in the development of interventions to address these needs.

In the interim, do not be surprised if you find that in facing this diagnosis, your usual ways of coping and handling problems don't seem to work for you. As you find new ways to deal with living with this diagnosis, look around for support groups run by reputable programs. Your urologist or oncologist may know of some. The ACOR listserv at www.acor.org can help you to find a support group. Psychologists and clinical social workers who help people deal with other cancers can be useful to you in helping you to realign your life. Asking for help is never a sign of weakness. A diagnosis of renal cell carcinoma can feel devastating. You do not have to face it alone.

NOTES:

NOTES:

CHAPTER 10
My Uncool, Quirky Cancer
by Susan Quella

My father was diagnosed with bilateral hypernephroma in 1956. I was fourteen at the time and wasn't told of his diagnosis or the seriousness of it. No one in the family was told, including my father. How different the medical environment was then. My mother, who was very strong-willed, told the doctors that she didn't want my father to know his devastating diagnosis, so they kept it a secret. For many years! That wouldn't happen now, thank God. But in 1956, they didn't tell this very intelligent bank president and community leader that he had cancer. They told him he had kidney disease. He would discuss it with family members—a couple of relatives who had guessed, and they had the uneasy task of not revealing it to him. I don't know if I could have passed it off.

My father's cancer had become very advanced by the time he became symptomatic and sought the advice of doctors. He was urinating bloody urine and had lost thirty-five pounds that he could not afford to lose. The surgeons quickly removed one kidney and treated the other kidney with cobalt radiation. He appeared terminally ill for several months, even to the point of periodically being in a light coma, then began to rally. Finally, he went back to work and that long medical crisis was forgotten by most of us. I graduated from high school and went away to college. My mother never said another word about it and my father said he had beaten "it".

In 1961, my father began getting quite ill again. He was such a stoic person that for months we didn't realize how much pain he was having. But soon he could no longer work and he would spend his days lying in bed, listening to the composers on the "hi-fi." I was in college across the country then and so full of myself that I never realized something was wrong at home. I never questioned why he didn't come to the phone when I called—until finally it was just too obvious in 1962 and I asked the question. That seemed to give my mother the impetus to say that my father was ill again and that I needed to come home and help. I was appalled when I saw him!

Those days when I was home helping take care of my father have given me such bittersweet memories. I would sit with him every day, caring for him, watching, frightened that he would breathe his last, and so proud of him for his strength. He would go in and out of what the doctors called uremic poisoning comas. The tiny portion of the remaining kidney that was working would become overwhelmed and not be able to filter out the body's waste products and he would go into the coma. After a few days, that little piece of kidney would kick in again and he would come out of it. Once, after being in a light coma for a few days, my father rolled over, looked at me, and said "What a difference a day makes!" He went on like this for another two years. By this time my mother had finally told him that he had cancer and the family, all had guessed it by then, didn't have to be so careful about letting the diagnosis slip. At the end, nine years after his initial diagnosis, and while he was saying that he was going to beat this thing yet, he died. The doctors said his body was full of cancer from head to toe.

In 2001, I awakened to my fourth episode of diverticulitis. I went to work bent over from the pelvic pain, running a fever of 102°, and having difficulty walking more than a few steps at a time. I knew what the diagnosis was because I'd experienced three previous episodes in the two proceeding years. Thinking I was so smart, I phoned my physician and told her I was experiencing another episode of diverticulitis and could she please call in an antibiotic "script" for me so that I could begin to treat myself.

Luckily, my physician is a lot smarter than I. She wanted to see me. I, of course, thought that I was too busy and would she please just call in a script and I would make a future appointment. She wanted to see me NOW! I had to trudge over to her office a block away, bent over and HOT! My physician called for an emergency CT scan, which, of course, showed severe, abscessed diverticulitis needing immediate surgical removal of that portion of the bowel, a gallbladder full of stones, a left kidney cyst and stones, and an incidental solid mass in my right kidney. Before she spoke, my physician held my hand, looked deep into my eyes and became very quiet. I knew that something really serious was about to be said.

The whole of my mind shattered into pieces to take on the many duties of listening, thinking, decision making, and feeling. One piece, my psyche, stepped outside of my body and the remainder of our conversation felt to me to be observed from outside of myself, instead of actually participating. I observed her telling me the diagnosis and the plan to take me into surgery in two days with two teams of surgeons, gastrointestinal and urologic. But my mind was going far beyond what she was telling me. My mind was telling me to remember the last two years of my father's life and how he had suffered. My mind told me to remember how my father was in so much pain, and how he had to sit at a 90° angle in a chair at all times because the metastatic tumors in his lungs and throat would cut off his air when he would lie back even 15°. My mind told me that I was just beginning to know my darling grandchildren and this was going to end up just like when I was a small child and all my grandparents were dead—and just like my daughter's childhood when my father died before they could know him. I wanted to "know" my grandchildren in every stage of their lives and have the chance to give them wonderful memories. I also thought that I needed to run home and get those twenty years worth of photos in all the new photo albums I've bought at sidewalk sales over the past years—and clean my closets because if I died soon, as I surely would, and if there was any conscious spirit after death, I wouldn't want to hear what my girls and their husbands would be saying about me while they were having to clean my closets!

I even thought how interesting it was that my physician could be sitting with me and I was hearing her talk, but I wasn't "with" her and had not been "with" her since the words "solid mass". I thought about dying. Would I be more fortunate than my father and die easily? Or, was suffering a family trait?

I thought that my two daughters were becoming such interesting, successful women and I wouldn't be here to participate in any way with their lives. They are also so much fun and I can't stand leaving them. Surely, it wouldn't be as much fun where I was going! That triggered thoughts about the concept of life after death. What did that mean? Does it mean the biblical concept of life after death or the spiritualist's concept of life after death? Would I just be stepping into another dimension? Would I be able to watch my family, see my grandchildren grow, watch them raise their families?

I remembered that my beloved sister and I had plans to travel over as much of the nation, and perhaps the world, as we could. We have had a few past adventures that have included frequent hysteria due to my directional dyslexia. Over the years, we have learned to be very calm when getting lost. No panic at all. In fact, we try to use it to our advantage and find something interesting about the place that has become our new destination. I thought about my wonderful friends. I have been so lucky to have friends that complete me so well. They have made my life so abundant and rich.

I don't remember being "integrated" again for several days. I don't remember the next day. I know from my records that I had an appointment with one of the top gastrointestinal surgeons in the institution and twelve inches of my bowel would be removed along with my gallbladder and appendix. I know that I was offered a clinical trial and I signed a consent form, but I don't think I took in anything about the trial. Thirty minutes after I signed the consent form, the resident came back in and told me that I didn't qualify because I didn't match one of the study's eligibility criteria and I became quite frightened that more was wrong than I knew and it was so advanced that I couldn't even be on a trial. He didn't explain.

What makes that so interesting to me is that I have been a cancer research nurse for twenty years and my area of expertise is the writing of consent forms in language that is understandable to patients of all walks of life and the importance of understanding what patients are going through at the time a cancer clinical trial is offered to a patient and how delicately and knowingly the "process" of consenting must be delivered. For twenty years, I have been giving presentations to the medical community, teaching residents, consultants, nurses, and research associates how important it is that they be on the same page as the patient because the patient is so traumatized by the diagnosis. I have repeatedly stressed to them that consenting must never be just a paper signing event, but a process throughout the relationship with the patient so that the professional is forever reminding the patient the what, why and wherefore of the trial they are being a partner in. I was exhibiting behavior that I described other patients going through, but at the time didn't even recognize it.

I also saw the urologist that next day. He was a friend, someone I had worked with for ten years earlier in my career. He is also known as a very aggressive kidney surgeon. I had personally witnessed this surgeon successfully removing extremely complicated tumors that had wrapped themselves around organs and body structures that left other urologic surgeons elsewhere in the country backing off and telling their patient that there was nothing they or anyone else could do to help them. Of course I would turn to him in my desperate need. I was still not "integrated" when I saw him, but vaguely remember that he said that once he removed this tumor, I would never see this cancer again! Hmmm, I must have a low stage tumor. I wonder if others had told me that. Probably.

The next thing I recall is that I am waiting in the lobby of the hospital and my daughters and son-in-laws are with me. I am to go up to the surgical floor in a few minutes. I don't know what I did the previous night. Did I call my daughters or did someone else, perhaps one of my friends, call them? I also don't remember them coming from their respective cities. I felt so numb; not really unhappy or terribly frightened, just numb. My eldest daughter started crying after we were escorted to the surgical floor and I was put in a room to change into a patient gown. To lighten the mood, as I was escorted down the hall to the preparation room and I left them behind, I mooned them. I walked in to be placed on a gurney with loud exclamations of disbelief behind me.

As I was lying on the gurney, knowing I was to be wheeled into the surgical suite in a few minutes, I tried to integrate so that I could be calm and adult when I was wheeled in. But, it was all so surreal. Four surgeons were about to cut me from stem to stern with two long incisions and take a portion of my right kidney out, clean my left kidney of its cyst and stones and take out a foot of bowel. As a nurse, I should remember how many feet that leaves me! But, when I became a patient, I stopped being a nurse! I knew I had to act as though I was a knowledgeable professional, but it would be an act. What if it's worse than they think and when they get inside me they realize I need a colostomy? What if they find metastatic renal cell carcinoma that didn't show up on the CT scan because it was lurking behind some structure? I can imagine bad things lurking in my body! Can I be as brave as my patients have been? And, how do they draw on that amazing spirit that cancer patients show us when they are going through rough times? I don't think I can be that strong.

Well—I finally "came to". I was finally integrated. It was the day after surgery and the nurses actually thought I would get out of bed and walk. The act of standing at my bedside was Herculean! And, they weren't satisfied with that! Amazing. There is nothing more effective to bring one around than pain. Numbness was gone. If I have described a normal reaction to this serious diagnosis, then the human organism is wired all wrong. One should have complete clarity when receiving a devastating diagnosis so that one can discuss options with their physicians and remember what was said and decided. Then, when they are experiencing mind-boggling pain, the numbness should kick in so that one doesn't feel it or at least remember it.

I was a floor nurse back in the 1960s. I well remember telling my surgical patients that the sooner they get out of bed, the easier their recovery will be. And I proved that to be true. I did so much walking during my post-operative period that I healed quickly and easily. However, I developed huge incisional hernias post-operatively, one in my right flank area and the other in the abdominal midline. The CT scans show the right flank hernia to have an absence of the overlying muscle and my liver hanging out into the hernia. My midline hernia has bowel resting in it. Did I do something wrong? Did a resident forget to pull the muscle back over the wound and stitch it in place? I'll never know.

I'm 62 years old and I look as though I'm carrying twins. I cannot look at myself in the mirror. The hernias are grotesque and disfiguring and whenever I mistakenly catch a glimpse of myself in a store window, my thought is that now I'm a physical freak. I have the pregnancy-like back pains and people do a second and third double-take when I am walking toward them. I tell them I'm due in a couple of weeks! I need to have another large surgery to repair the hernias and I keep putting it off. For one thing, the repairs don't usually hold and I've known cases of patients having two or three surgeries. For another, my insurance won't pay for what they describe as cosmetic surgery. I'm in pain. I can't wear normal dresses anymore. I can't lie on my stomach. I can't have a massage. I will not put on a swimsuit—ever again! And, I have to be very careful not to bump my liver. They still think that's cosmetic surgery! But, I'm alive. My father died at age sixty-two of this disease and I'm alive. Not much else is as important as that! Inhale....

My philosophy has changed so very much, about almost everything. I was a driven career woman, working twelve hour days, trying to find answers to research questions. I also felt compelled to join many efforts to teach, help, advise at my institution and in Washington D.C. My house was clean, my garden weeded. Now, I have taken an early retirement and am attempting to start a consulting business in my home. I used to awaken at 5:15 A.M. without the assist of an alarm. Now I'm awakening at 7:30 A.M. I can sit at my computer on my time, with my amazing mini-dachshund sitting next to me, and be accountable only to myself. I thought I would work for my employer until at least age 70, but that perspective has completely changed. I am now reducing the stress in my life in as many areas as possible. I sit in the glider and watch the birds at least a couple afternoons a week. Last week I took a class in European flower tying and another in silver jewelry making. Next week it is to be a class on centerpiece arranging. I look into my garden and there are weeds almost as tall as I. Maybe I'll get out there and battle with them tomorrow. But, maybe I won't. For the first time in my life, I have a stack of dishes in my kitchen sink. I know this is a reaction to what I have been through and knowing my personality, I will get my act together soon. I will also gradually add more serious efforts. But, I will have learned how to balance them more effectively.

Since my cancer experience, I have been a member of an international renal cell carcinoma listserv. There is some disadvantage to being a member of a cancer listserv. The most prominent downside is that one can get very addicted to spending each day reading about what others are going through with this disease. I was checking in two or three times a day and getting so caught-up in the lives and struggles of others. And, in time, some of the frequent contributors have eventually been considered my friends. When one experiences a recurrence, I become frightened for them. It makes the possibility of recurrence more real for me and I become frightened for me also. When one loses the struggle, I mourn deeply. To stave off being overwhelmed by the pain and losses, I finally have had to strictly curtail my activity on the listserv.

An additional downside has been to learn how unenlightened our insurance companies and Medicare have become. I have so much difficulty understanding how they can turn down paying for their clients' cancer tests and treatments, including clinical trials. When did we become such a callused world? I continually read about patients who have paid premiums for years, only to get this devastating disease and have to battle their insurance companies to get them to pay for their healthcare. Some of them are so ill, yet they have to spend hours trying to work with their insurance companies.

On the other hand, there are many positive aspects to being a member of the listserv. One is the sense of community, as the definition of community being a unified body of individuals. Throughout life, one moves through many life communities. Initially it is the family. Then one becomes part of an academic community. One becomes part of a community of friends. Also the work environment becomes a community. For some, church becomes a community for them. Community is safe and one has a sense of belonging, of purpose, of "home". Having a diagnosis of cancer separates us from people, even those who are closest to us. It just can't be changed. We are the ones with the disease. Even though our family and friends commiserate with us, love us, and help us as much as they can, we are the ones who are afraid. We are the ones who are in pain. We are the ones who are facing the tests, the treatments and the mortality issues. Even though they can walk beside us, no-one can take that journey for us. The listserv members are also on the journey and they, more than anyone, can understand.

Another positive aspect of being an active member of a listserv is altruistic of course. It is fulfilling to be able to help another who is struggling. Often, I will write one of the members "off-list" to offer them support, advice on nursing care or sadly and too often, condolences. The caregivers of affected family members write asking why their loved one is experiencing certain symptoms and I can send them information of known side effects of drugs their loved one is taking or to just give them encouragement.

There are so many inspiring, giving people on the listserv who are either patients fighting amazingly hard to conquer or at least control this disease, or family members and friends fighting so hard to keep their patient healthy or at best, symptom free.

Listserv membership gives members an amazing amount of knowledge about renal cell carcinoma, treatments, trials, legislation, who and where the experts are, and how to access it all. Every listserv member, who learns something new, rushes to get it on the listserv so that all may benefit. Many listserv members attend national cancer conferences and listen to the experts. Many research their diagnosis and the treatment options diligently. Many talk to their oncologists and write their conversations down for us all. I am constantly amazed at their level of knowledge.

I have learned so much more about renal cell carcinoma than I'd ever learned as a nurse, in the books or on the floor. The most absolute lesson has been to be ever vigilant, even if it was a low stage cancer. My urologist has not seen me since my first post-op visit nine weeks after surgery. At that time he again stated that I would not see this cancer in the future. I really want to believe him, but what about all the stage I or II patients that I read about on the listserv that experience devastating recurrences?

Since my renal cell carcinoma diagnosis, I have developed a few benign dermatofibromas on my arms and legs and have had plastic surgeons remove them and send them to pathology to have them checked out. Why is it that those physicians tell me that it's wise being vigilant because renal cell carcinoma is "quirky", but my urologist has said I don't need to have any follow-up? I have read the statistics of low grade renal cell carcinoma recurring and it is low. Many urologists believe that there is not a need for much follow-up if one has a low grade tumor. But what if I am one of the low number of patients that does experience a recurrence? It is better to find it early!

Another lesson I have learned is that not only patients but also many physicians are not up to date on what treatments are considered the treatment of choice currently; or how appropriately aggressive some surgeons are becoming with this disease, saving people instead of writing them off; or what clinical trials are being offered and where. I can see how this happens. Oncologists not involved with a large teaching medical center don't have time to go to conferences, read all the journals that come out every month, or talk with the experts frequently. Almost every cancer is increasing in incidence and these physicians are just too busy. We need to change the way information is dispersed. Maybe it would help to have e-mail news-flashes sent out frequently—short, forceful, instructive briefs with a reference attached so that the physician can look it up when he or she has time.

The third thing I know is that there are not enough researchers interested in renal cell carcinoma and not nearly enough research dollars. Renal cell carcinoma is diagnosed in over 30,000 people per year and has a five-year survival rate of about 55%. These are not heartening statistics. Even though renal cell carcinoma is increasing in incidence each year, research funds are not increasing in proportion. There's also a huge discrepancy between what is offered for other cancers and what is offered for renal cell research. I am finding an amazing lack of interest in this diagnosis which is causing me to become an activist for renal cell research. I have begun to watch how congress is spending their research dollars and writing to congressmen urging them to release more funds for renal cell research. I'm also becoming more daring in questioning oncologists about their involvement, or lack of, in renal cell research.

I have had a cancer that is not popular. It makes me feel like I did when I was a teenager and the "clique" of girls that I wanted to be associated with would shun me because I wasn't "cool" enough. Now, I have an uncool cancer! I feel such a sense of disbelief. Why are there some cancers that are so popular to fight for and some that are not? And, why does it have to become both a social and a political issue, besides a medical one? Does it make any difference if I write to my congressman? Some of them don't even answer me and the ones that do send me preprinted "thank you for your interest" notes. Is this what they mean by the power of one? I think not. But, just in case, I'll keep writing—and talking to people about the importance of renal cell carcinoma research funding. I have joined a national patient advocacy group who is teaching me how to become an effective crusader.

For this chapter, I was asked to write what my experiences have been since being diagnosed with renal cell carcinoma. Initially, I didn't think I had anything to say, but as you can see, that diagnosis has been a life-altering experience for me. The diagnosis of cancer changes everyone—our perspective on who we are and what our world will be like from then on is radically altered. We move into another community.

NOTES:

NOTES:

CHAPTER 11

State-of-the-Art Immunotherapeutic Approaches to Treat Kidney Cancer

by Eugene D. Kwon, M.D.

For many decades now, both physicians and scientists have worked together to try to coax the human immune system to unleash an attack against the various forms of malignancy that afflict patients. Such malignancies include cancers of the kidney, lungs, liver, skin, colon, bladder, prostate, and breast and ovaries. In short, these efforts have encompassed an extremely long and arduous journey to identify various methods to manipulate human immune cells so that these immune cells would be capable of *identifying* and then *attacking* patient tumor cells so as to induce tumor cell death and regression in response to a toxic attack by the immune system. In this chapter, much attention will be directed towards T lymphocytes which are regarded as the primary immune cells that are responsible for attacking tumor cells by virtue of their ability to recognize tumor cells, bind to tumor cells and then to inject toxic substances into tumor cells so as to cause their demise. Thus, in layman's terms, the primary goal of cancer immunotherapy is to generate a potent host immune response that is ultimately capable of causing tumor regression in the clinical setting. And the host immune response that is desired specifically pertains to a response by T lymphocytes that are regarded as the "primary fighters" of the immune system against cancer.

Now an obvious question is, "why would the human immune system be regarded as something that is capable of killing tumors or various forms of human malignancy?" The answer to this question is fairly straightforward. For instance, for a long time now it has been recognized that the human immune system can be manipulated using vaccines to wage war against various pathogens such as bacteria as well as viruses so as to prevent disease onset and progression in patients. Vaccination of the human immune system has been resoundingly successful in preventing disease onset and progression against a number of illnesses that emanate from either bacterial or virus infection. For instance, we now have effective vaccines that have, in essence, either eradicated or prevented widespread outbreaks of various diseases that were once very common including polio, pertussis, diphtheria, rubella, small pox, measles, mumps and tetanus. Many of these vaccines have been developed within our lifetime and it is within our lifetime that we have seen many of these diseases bow to the success of scientific discovery and translation into the clinical setting. Related to this, it should be realized that the process of "vaccination" typically involves using a piece or a portion of either a bacterium or virus and then inactivating that piece of the bacterium or virus using various approaches. Subsequently that moiety is then injected into a patient. Following injection of bacterial or viral fragments or "antigens" into the patient, the patient's immune system becomes aware and educated to identify the pathogen. In response to this, various immune cells then expand (multiply) within the patient and their activity becomes heightened so that they may aggressively roam and survey the body in the event that a certain pathogen enters into the body. Upon entry of a given bacterium or virus, antigen-educated immune cells (which are typically T cells or T lymphocytes) identify and attack "anything" that bears portions of the virus or bacteria on its surface, including virus or bacterium that has just entered the body to initiate a disease process.

In addition to being a good thing, the human immune system can be a terribly bad thing when it goes awry. A number of autoimmune diseases are known to be disorders where immune cells within the patient run amuck, attacking normal tissues in the body, thereby causing disease. For instance, disorders such as Multiple Sclerosis, Scleroderma, Systemic Lupus Erythematosus (SLE), Type I Diabetes, Crohn's disease, and Rheumatoid Arthritis are all manifestations of a faulty human immune system attacking normal tissues within the body. In fact, there are roughly 70 other syndromes that are caused by the immune system going awry and attacking normal tissues within the body. In addition to this, it is the human immune system that is the bad guy in the context of organ rejection following transplantation. For instance, when a kidney, or a liver, or a heart, or a lung, or a pancreas is rejected following transplant, it is the human immune system that is mediating the rejection of that organ. Therefore, most patients that receive transplants must be "immuno-suppressed" in order to prevent their own immune system from destroying the otherwise "foreign" transplanted organ. Autoimmune disease as well as transplant organ rejection both underscore the power of the human immune system, demonstrating that the human immune system — when triggered — is capable of destroying huge organs or tissues to the point that those organs or tissues are no longer viable. Related to this, there are many other diseases or processes that also underscore how powerful the human immune system can be. For instance, if a patient receives an injury to one eye, in 10% of those patients, the uninjured eye may be attacked by an immune response or even rejected and, thus, the patient may go blind. The reason that this occurs is because there are various parts of the eye or antigens that are sequestered from the human immune system, and when they are revealed to the human immune system they act like a vaccine causing an immune response to target normal parts of the eye. Consequently, in subsets of patients who injure one eye, the normal uninjured eye is also attacked by immune inflammation causing a form of bilateral blindness, a dramatic and extreme result of the immune system gone terribly awry. Similar to this, some patients that receive a bite injury from a brown recluse spider will also subsequently generate an immune response against their own skin. This response can sometimes occur even many, many months after the initial brown recluse spider bite, causing large portions of the skin to slough entirely from the backs or arms of patients who have been bitten by the brown recluse spider. In summary, the human immune system can be a powerfully good or bad thing. At any rate, it is clear that the human immune system is capable of causing massive destruction of either abnormal or even normal tissues when it is manipulated and educated to attack these tissues.

Another obvious question is "why after all of these years do we suddenly now think that we can get T lymphocytes or T cells to identify and then destroy cancer?" The answer to this is that within the last several years, we and others have learned how to precisely coax or educate T cells to fight against cancer. Specifically, it has been within the last 10 to 15 years that we have learned that T cells actually attack normal and abnormal cells based on a number of signals that they receive from those cells. Within the last 10 years it has become extremely clear that T lymphocytes require two signals in order to become activated in a "specific" fashion so that these T cells can then go on to attack tumors to cause their destruction. It should be noted that there are many different "flavors" of T cells that float around the body. Some of these T cells are referred to as CD8 T cells whereas others are referred to as CD4 T cells. CD8 T cells typically are the ones that are responsible for grabbing on to a tumor cell or a cellular target to promote killing of that cell by actually binding to that cell and injecting toxins into that cell. CD4 T cells, on the other hand, tend to be either "helpers" or "inhibitors" in that they can influence the response of the CD8 T cell by providing the CD8 T cell with various signals that either turn them on or off. In reference to the two signals that are required to turn T cells on, the T cells must first make contact with an "antigen" or a portion of the tumor cell so that it can identify the tumor cell and then bind to it. It has become extremely clear, however, that the antigen alone is not sufficient to turn a T cell on. In fact, a T cell not only requires an antigen, but also requires a second signal in order to be fully activated. The second signal is referred to as a "costimulatory signal", and when an antigen and a costimulatory signal is provided to the T cell, the T cell then turns on and is capable of moving on to the next step of activation. Now it should be noted that there are roughly a billion different forms of T cells floating around in the body, each with its own receptor to identify a specific antigen. Upon recognizing the antigen and receiving the important second "costimulatory signal", the T cell is then able to multiply or "clone" itself, creating an army of T cells that are specific against any one particular antigen. It is at that point that an army of T cells must be generated so that a successful war against a tumor or tumor cells can be initiated. Within the last five years there have been a number of important discoveries that make it even clearer how a given T cell can make the stepwise succession into an army of T cells. Following T cell activation by the two signals, it is now clear that T cells additionally will manufacture a number of additional molecules and receptors that can either further turn the T cell on, or, perhaps more importantly, turn the T cell off entirely. Such molecules and receptors include cytokines such as Interleukin 2 (IL-2), Interferon gamma (IFN-α), and granulocyte- macrophage colony stimulating factor (GM-CSF). In addition following costimulatory activation, T cells also will decorate themselves with a number of receptors such as the 4-1BB, ICOS, OX-40, CTLA-4, and the PD-1 receptor. These receptors are fascinating in that some of these receptors further turn T cells on, whereas other receptors turn T cells off again. For instance, 4-1BB, ICOS, the IL-2 receptor, and the OX-40 receptor, are all responsible for causing T cells to become even more activated, thereby energizing them so that they can wage a more productive war against tumors. In contrast, some of the receptors such as the CTLA-4 receptor, the PD-1 receptor, and the B7-H1 molecule — when they are engaged — act as inhibitors to turn a T cell off again. In fact, some of these inhibitory receptors, when engaged, will not only inhibit the T cell but also kill it and completely remove it from the immune system. Now the question is, "why would nature build such powerful switches into T cells to cause them to turn on or turn off?"

The answer to this is quite obvious. Nature intended to provide a very tightly-regulated safety-mechanism so that T cells can be turned off again when the inflammatory response needs to be stopped or aborted for whatever reason. For example, if you develop an infection and T cells are appearing at the site of inflammation and the pathogenic process or insult is then cleared, nature must have a means whereby to turn those T cells off again, otherwise you would suffer from a chronically festering wound or process. Similarly, T cells gone awry must be turned off as quickly as possible so that they do not wage an accidental war against normal host tissues, thereby causing autoimmune disorder. Related to that, it is clear that some autoimmune processes such as rheumatoid arthritis, multiple sclerosis, etc., in fact, are a consequence of the inability to stop T cell responses.

At any rate, it is the multitude of these very recent discoveries of the T cell receptors and molecules that govern T cells activation and inactivation that provide the basis for the most current forms of immunotherapy that are being used or exploited to treat cancer in patients. For instance, at the present time there are many investigators who are now using various manipulations of the T cell receptors so that the patient's T cells can become more potent, thereby fighting a more productive war against cancer. Specifically, antibodies and molecules directed against the "go" signals for the T cell such IL-2, 4-1BB, and ICOS, OX-40 have all been generated so that the patient may be injected with antibodies to provide these critical "go" signals to stimulate T cells that can be directed against tumors, thereby evoking more rapid tumor regression. Many of these antibodies are currently either being developed or produced and tested in clinical phase I, II, and III trials. Some of the responses that have been observed using these T cell "go" signal antibodies, have been so profound that — for the first time ever — we have observed complete tumor regression in various animal models harboring relatively large tumors. In addition, in the clinical setting, some of these antibodies and molecules have demonstrated the ability to potentiate or stimulate the immune system to the point where partial or complete tumor regression is observed. One of the most extensively tested immune molecules for the treatment of advanced kidney cancer is IL-2. IL-2 has been applied with varying degrees of success against advanced kidney cancer. In fact, high dose IL-2 therapy is considered, in some regards, a standard form of therapy to treat patients with advanced forms of kidney cancer. In subsets of advanced kidney cancer patients — roughly 10 to 15% of these patients — a response is typically observed which is either transient or prolonged. However, it is also clear that IL-2 therapy alone is typically insufficient to cause complete tumor regression for the lifetime of the patient. Associated with this, it has been demonstrated that IL-2 therapy is moderately toxic and, thus, there is great interest in developing other immune therapies that can be combined with IL-2 therapy to reduce the toxicity of IL-2 therapy while also improving the anti-tumor response than is elicited during immunotherapeutic treatment. Many of these adjunctive manipulations will include manipulations of the other accessory - costimulatory ("go") molecules that activate T cells such as 4-1BB, ICOS and OX-40.

Related to all of this, it has further been demonstrated that in order to turn on a T cell with the two signals, one may use something called an antigen-presenting cell (APC) which typically is decorated with the exact two signals that are required to turn on a T cell. The antigen-presenting cell is much like a scavenger fish that one sees at the bottom of a fish tank. Antigen-presenting cells such as activated B cells, dendritic cells, macrophages and monocytes typically roam around the body and scour up or scavenge antigens from dying or injured cells that are residing within the host. Once they have scavenged these antigens, they typically decorate their surface with these antigens and, under certain circumstances, also decorate themselves with costimulatory molecules (B7.1, B7.2), thereby obtaining the capability to provide the critical two signals that are essential to evoke T cell activation. Thus there has been great interest in using antigen-presenting cells that have been stuffed full of tumor antigens as a means to vaccinate the immune system to cause T cell activation against tumors. So one can clearly envision how antigen-presenting cells may be useful as an initial vaccine to treat tumors. One can also envision how other co-accessory or costimulatory molecules may be manipulated to then take APC-activated T cells in order to drive them further forward to mount and sustain a meaningful anti-tumor response.

As mentioned before, however, T cells will simultaneously generate a number of stop receptors or stop signals on their surface following costimulatory activation. These stop signals include signals emanating from the receptor for CTLA-4, the receptor for PD-1 as well as the molecule B7-H1. What is interesting about these molecules is that it has been clearly demonstrated that if you block these stop signals, a T cell may be permitted to move forward and continue to clone itself and proliferate and attack tumor cells in an highly aggressive fashion. Hence, there has been enormous interest to generate various antibodies and molecules that will block CTLA-4, PD-1 and B7-H1 to permit T cells to move forward in an unfettered fashion so that they may aggressively attack tumor cells. In fact, many of these molecules have now been generated and are being tested in clinical phase I, II, and III trials. Specifically, an antibody directed against the CTLA-4 receptors has now been generated and provided for clinical use. Anti-CTLA-4 has been extensively tested against melanoma and, in fact, is being tested against a number of other cancers as well including prostate cancer, breast cancer, and kidney cancer. What is interesting is that patients that receive the antibody against CTLA-4 have been demonstrated to mount an immune response against their cancers. Sometimes the response can be modest, but at other times, the response can be so potent that not only does one observe tumor regression but also rejection of normal tissues that are associated with that tumor. For instance in melanoma — which is a cancer of the cells that produce the dark pigment within the skin — patients with melanoma that have been treated with anti-CTLA-4 antibody sometimes will additionally demonstrate loss of pigmentation in their skin as well as other sites of the body including the retinas of their eyes. This illustrates how potent of an immune response can be unleashed when the stop signals to the immune system are suddenly blocked. In other words, blocking the stop signals to the immune signals can, in some regards, be akin to removing the brakes from an automobile, thereby causing the automobile to move forward with no mechanism of stopping. Nevertheless, the ability to remove inhibitory signals to T cells constitutes one of the most important discoveries for immunotherapeutic treatment in recent times. In fact, it is quite clear that in order to unleash a favorable anti-tumoral response against kidney cancer, as well as other forms of malignancies, it will be very critical to remove these inhibitory signals at the proper time during immunotherapeutic treatment. Related to this, it is important to note that a very, very powerful inhibitory molecule called B7-H1 has now been discovered to be demonstrated in great abundance on the surface of kidney cancer cells. B7-H1 on the tumor cells is known to interact with the T cell receptor, PD-1. B7-H1 on kidney tumor cells then interacts with T cell PD-1 to cause T cells to die. In other words, B7-H1 on the surface of kidney cancer cells acts like barbed wire, popping any T cells that come near the kidney tumor cell. It is this mechanism that is currently believed to protect kidney cancer cells from attack by T cells or host immune cells. Our group has recently demonstrated that the more B7-H1 that is present on the surface of the tumor cell, the more likely the kidney cancer is going to progress and cause death in the patient with the tumor that expresses B7-H1. These results are the first demonstration ever of an immune molecule participating in or mediating the progression of a solid cancer. In addition, our observations basically reveal a very promising strategy to disarm kidney cancer cells so that the human immune system can then participate by attacking the kidney tumor and, thus, causing its rejection and destroying any associated metastases. Specifically, our group is currently working on strategies to block B7-H1 on the surface of kidney tumor cells so that the patient's immune system can more freely approach the tumor cells to cause their regression and destruction. This strategy, in many regards, is analogous to putting a rubber tip on the end of a sharp lance so that it can no longer inflict any penetrating damage. Hence, the strategy that we envision — and one that has now been extensively tested in the experimental setting — is via the use of an antibody that will bind to the surface of kidney tumor cells that display B7-H1. By doing so, T cells will be permitted to readily enter kidney tumors and destroy the tumor cells. The importance of this approach is three-fold. First of all, we have now demonstrated that B7-H1 represents a very important marker for the aggressiveness of a kidney tumor. In fact, B7-H1 can be used to predict, with a moderate amount of accuracy, which patients are most likely to have spread of their cancer as well as experience an increased risk of death from their cancer. Thus, B7-H1 functions as a prognostic marker for kidney cancer. In addition, we believe that B7-H1 may be useful to determine which patients are most likely to respond to the various forms of systemic immunotherapy that are generally available to treat advanced kidney cancer including IL-2 or INF-α cytokine therapy for extensive kidney cancer. Finally, we are extremely encouraged by the fact that B7-H1 may represent one of these most promising targets for the treatment of aggressive kidney carcinoma. At present, we believe that by blocking B7-H1 expression on the surface of kidney tumor cells, we may be able to then render those tumors much more responsive to other forms of therapy including immunotherapy, thereby eliciting either a complete response or one that is more durable for patients with extensive kidney cancer. The importance of B7-H1, however, extends far beyond kidney cancer. In fact, we also now know that B7-H1 is expressed on the surface of many different forms of cancer including bladder, breast, cervical, colon, endometrial, gallbladder, brain, head and neck, liver, lung, ovarian, kidney, stomach, thyroid and thymic cancers as well as lymphoma, melanoma and mesothelioma. From this we infer that by inhibiting or blocking B7-H1 on the surface of these tumors, we may be able to improve the treatment of all of these cancers as well. However, at the present time further studies will be necessary in order to determine whether or not B7-H1 blockade will be useful to improve treatment of these various cancers.

With regards to kidney cancer, it should also be pointed out that there is currently a plethora of new approaches to treat kidney cancer using an immunotherapeutic approach. Such approaches include cytokine therapy, adjunctive therapy, dendritic cell therapy, the use of antigenic vaccines, manipulations of the co-stimulatory or co-inhibitory receptors on the surface of T cells, monoclonal antibody therapy as well as removal (depletion) of certain T lymphocytes that participate in inhibiting immune responses against kidney cancer. For instance, as alluded to previously, many investigators are exploring the use of dendritic cells as antigen-presenting cells in order to vaccinate patients against kidney cancer. Dendritic cells, as mentioned before, are like scavenger cells that survey the body and vacuum up antigen from dead and dying cells. Because antigen-presenting cells (APC's) or dendritic cells can then decorate themselves with the antigen and present the antigen to T lymphocytes along with costimulatory molecules such as B7.1 or B7.2, these APCs or dendritic cells are very potent at activating T lymphocytes in order to induce a response against kidney cancer. In most current scenarios, dendritic cells are removed from the patient and then expanded in laboratory dishes so that an abundance of dendritic cells can be infused back into the patient in order to evoke an immune response against the patient's tumor. In many of these situations, during the laboratory expansion phase, the dendritic cells are also either genetically re-engineered or stuffed full of kidney tumor antigens so that they may evoke a powerful response against kidney tumors. In fact, dendritic cells are widely being explored as a possible form of vaccine in many clinical phase I, II, and III trials. Beyond this, dendritic cells have also been artificially fused to kidney tumor cells so that the kidney tumor cells can manufacture antigens that are directly then used by the dendritic cell to be presented on its surface to evoke T cell activation against kidney tumors. This form of cell is called a hybridoma in which dendritic cells are actually fused to a kidney tumor cell so that it is half "antigen-presenting" and half tumor cell. These hybridomas are then injected back into the patient so that they may present abundant antigen to the patient's T cells so that it can readily recognize a kidney tumor cell and then attack it to cause tumor rejection.

Another scenario is the use of antigens that have been derived from tumor cells in order to create vaccines that can be then injected into the host patient to evoke a powerful response against kidney tumors. Such antigens can be generated by taking tumor cells and simply grinding them up and then re-infusing them back into the patient. Alternatively, kidney antigens can be incorporated into dendritic cells and then injected back into the patient as mentioned above. One set of antigen vaccines that has recently been created has been generated from heat-shock proteins. Heat shock proteins are proteins that are abundantly manufactured by normal as well as cancerous cells to act as scaffolds for all of the major proteins or molecules that are within the cell. These scaffolding heat-shock proteins protect the interior of normal and cancerous cells from various forms of stress including heat, cold and pressure. Thus, by purifying these heat-shock proteins from tumor cells, one can obtain a large repertoire of tumor antigens that can then be processed and re-injected into the patient as a vaccine so that the patient sees a broad repertoire of antigens that entirely represents the kidney tumor cells thereby raising a powerful T cell response which then can be mounted to attack kidney tumors. Such heat shock protein vaccines have now entered clinical testing and, at present, we are awaiting results of a phase III clinical trial using heat shock protein vaccines for the treatment of kidney cancer.

As alluded to before, a number of co-accessory or costimulatory antibodies have also been generated which act to provide potent "go" signals to T cells so that they can become more powerful to fight against kidney cancer. Such co-accessory or costimulatory antibodies includes those that target 4-1BB, OX-40, and ICOS which promote T cell activation, T cell multiplication, and T cell targeting of kidney cancers. Also mentioned before, a number of antibodies or molecules have been generated to block co-inhibitory receptors on the surface of T cells that are involved in shutting down T cell responses such as B7-H1 and CTLA-4 so that the T cell may function unimpeded to attack tumor cells to cause their complete regression. All of these co-accessory or costimulatory antibodies are now currently in clinical testing and the results of these tests are widely anticipated. At present most of these clinical trials are revealing very promising results.

In addition to these manipulations, there has been the very recent discovery of something called a T regulatory cell or "Treg cell" which is a certain flavor of T cell that functions to shut down other T cells. In other words, there is a specific subset of T cells that singularly functions to roam around the body to shut off other T cells, either by killing them or inhibiting their function. These Treg cells function by directly making contact with other T cells and then providing them with signals that cause target T cells to fail. Based on this, it is now widely recognized that by removing Treg cells from the blood stream, one might be able to enhance responses by other T cells that are capable of causing tumor regression, including regression of kidney cancer. Related to this, there have been a number of compounds that have been designed and generated to target Treg cells to remove them from the patient's circulation. One such compound employs a toxin that has been fused to IL-2 which then binds to Treg cells so that these Treg cells can be targeted and then killed while within the body. By doing so, it is expected that Treg cells will be removed from circulation, thereby letting other T cells function in an unfettered fashion to cause tumor regression.

In addition, a number of cytokines have been demonstrated to activate the immune system so that one gets a more powerful response against various tumors including kidney cancer. Such cytokines include IL-2, INF-α, and GM-CSF. All of these cytokines have been demonstrated to enhance immune responses against tumors such as kidney cancer to facilitate the regression of these kidney tumors, or other tumors as well, in the clinical setting. Most of these cytokines are now being explored in combination with other forms of immunotherapy such as dendritic cell vaccination or heat shock protein vaccination or blockade of inhibitory signaling so as to generate a robust response against kidney tumors in the clinical setting.

It has also been demonstrated that T lymphocytes within the body are vulnerable to being overcrowded and thus, being unable to function optimally. The analogy would be that of urban blight in which a certain urban population is overpopulated and, therefore, unable to function optimally. Based on this, it has recently been recognized that by removing various T cells from the body — using agents such as those employed during chemotherapeutic treatment — one can free-up space within the body so that new T cells can be generated, and during that process of regeneration, steered or directed towards tumors so as to evoke a potent anti-tumoral response. Some of the most promising data to date with regards to tumor immunotherapy has emanated from the National Cancer Institute in which patients have been treated with agents such as chemotherapy to removed their old, dysfunctional and somewhat "bureaucratic" T cells in order to create space for new T cells that can actively participate in an anti-tumoral response. In fact, in clinical trials it has been demonstrated that by removing old T cells from the body, one may be able to then vaccinate the patient using a variety of vaccine approaches combined with cytokine therapy in order to evoke a very potent anti-tumoral response which can cause complete tumor regression in the setting of advanced cancer. Some of these responses have been very complete and have occurred in melanoma patients that have failed all other forms of cancer treatment.

Related to this, it is important to recognize that it is very unlikely that a single form of immunotherapy is going to result in a complete response for a patient with advanced cancer. In light of this, it is thought that immunotherapy will likely be most efficacious for the patient when combined with other forms of immunotherapy or when given as a component of a multi-modality therapeutic approach. For instance, one can envision using vaccines and cytokines and monoclonal antibodies and various adjuvants as well as other immunotherapeutic manipulations all in combination in order to evoke a very potent anti-tumoral response. Similarly, it is envisioned that immunotherapy may be very useful when given after a surgical procedure which would be intended to remove the bulk of a tumor, or after radiation or chemotherapy or other non-immunotherapeutic forms of intervention have been rendered. Overall, it has been demonstrated that immunotherapy is very effective for small residual deposits of cancer that may be left behind following other forms of therapy given the fact that the immune system has a finite capacity to fight against tumors. Thus it is probably most optimal to treat residual cancer following other forms of intervention. Also, one must recognize that immunotherapy has several different potential applications. One is to prevent tumors before they form. Such prevention strategies would encompass a prophylactic vaccination to prevent the occurrence of tumors in patients before they have a chance to form and become established. Other applications of tumor immunotherapy include vaccination to eradicate tumors that are already present within the patient. As alluded to above, vaccination may also be useful to treat metastatic forms of cancer because the immune system is not localized to one part of the body but, in fact, roams the body and is able to fight cancer wherever it is encountered within the body. Thus, there is great enthusiasm to generate immunotherapeutic strategies to target metastases, especially in light of the fact that most forms of treatment for metastatic disease have only a limited application. As mentioned before, immunotherapy may be very useful to destroy residual cancer after a primary attempt to remove a large tumor that has already demonstrated microscopic spread to other environments within the body. Related to all of this, it is very important to recognize that kidney cancer is regarded as one of the most favorable targets for immunotherapeutic treatment. This perspective has been fostered by the observation that under some situations metastatic forms of kidney cancer disappear following removal of the primary tumor. The reason for this has long been speculated as being due to the triggering of an immune response that is capable of attacking metastases following removal of the primary kidney tumor. In addition, as is well recognized, kidney cancer has been demonstrated to be responsive to treatment with various cytokines that are known to influence the immune response of the host. Such cytokines include IL-2, INF-a, as well as GM-CSF.

In summary, scientists and physicians have made a number of observations that have educated researchers how to more precisely manipulate the immune system to target kidney cancer. These observations are very recent, very exciting and extend great promise for the development of immunotherapeutic strategies to treat kidney cancer as well as a number of other cancers. Among these observations include the observation of a very potent inhibitor of immune responses, B7-H1, which is displayed on the surface of kidney cancers. B7-H1 is a potent predictor of kidney cancer progression and death due to kidney cancer. In addition, B7-H1 encompasses a very favorable target for therapy. It is anticipated that by blocking B7-H1 expression on the surface of kidney tumors, one may be able to potentiate or facilitate immune responses that can then subsequently function to cause kidney cancer rejection or to facilitate responses to other forms of therapy. In terms of future directions, it is widely anticipated that a number of new molecules will be discovered that will further add to the overall armamentarium for immunotherapeutic intervention. In addition, it is widely anticipated that further phase I, II, and III clinical trial testing of these various forms of immunotherapy — either alone or in combination with other forms of immunotherapy or other forms of treatment such as surgery, radiation, or chemotherapy — will reveal robust strategies to treat advanced forms of kidney cancer more effectively. In short, the development of immunotherapeutic strategies for the treatment of kidney cancer encompasses one of the most exciting areas in science and medicine to date. It is with great hope and great anticipation that robust and highly efficacious forms of therapies for kidney cancer will soon be developed to make kidney cancer a "bad-dream" of our past.

Incidental
Finding

NOTES:

Resources

Your most important asset is YOU. No one else is as motivated as you and your loved ones to marshal the best resources to your aid. It is poignant that just when you are feeling most vulnerable you must engage most avidly and actively on your own behalf. I hope that this list will help you with that task, saving vital energy for your encounter with renal cell carcinoma. This is a basic list of resources. It is not meant to be comprehensive although using some of these resources will quickly link you to others. A blank page is included so that you may add your own resources as you discover them. Good Luck!

Special Note

The most important, useful first step you can take is to go to Steve Dunn's website, **www.cancerguide.org**. This website is a guide map for understanding kidney cancer and knowledgeably initiating and managing your own care. Steve Dunn was a Stage IV (terminal) kidney cancer patient who had been completely cured of kidney cancer 15 years before dying on August 19, 2005, from complications of bacterial meningitis. Steve's commitment to educating and supporting kidney cancer patients was exemplary.

ListServs and Chats

Kidney cancer listserv at **www.acor.org**
Chat room at **www.curekidneycancer.org**
Live chats with physicians at **www.plwc.org**

Websites (listed alphabetically)

The Association of Cancer Online Resources
– www.acor.org provides information and support to cancer patients
and those who care for them through the creation and maintenance
of cancer-related Internet mailing lists and Web-based resource.

American Cancer Society
– www.cancer.org website of the American Cancer Society

American Urological Association
– http://www.urologyhealth.org/adult/index.cfm?cat=04&topic=124
--provides basic information augmented by excellent illustrations

Birt Hogg Dube Alliance 1-877-764-4907
– www.birthoggdube.org is a source of information and contact for
those who are affected by or interested in the genetic Birt Hogg Dube,
or Birt-Hogg-Dube, syndrome.

Cancer Care, Inc.
– www.cancercare.org offers free support, information, financial
assistance and web linkages. Telephone 1-800-813-4673

Cancer Consultants Oncology Resource Center
– www.patient.cancerconsultants.com provides access to current
information about the screening, prevention, and treatment of
cancer by cancer type.

Cancer Guide
– www.cancerguide.org has in-depth information about kidney
cancer and helps you learn how to find the answers to your
questions, especially what questions you need to ask.

CancerLynx
– www.cancerlynx.com an online zine for cancer patients and
professionals–type "kidney cancer" into the search box for
excellent article by Robin Martinez.

Cancer Quest
– www.cancerquest.org does an excellent job of teaching the biology of
cancer. While no assumptions have been made about prior knowledge
of biology or cancer, the site does not "talk down" to lay readers.

Center for Patient Partnerships
– http://www.law.wisc.edu/patientadvocacy/index.html
  — works to empower patients as equal partners with providers
  to achieve successful health care outcomes.

Coalition of Cancer Trials Cooperative Groups
– www.cancertrialshelp.org provides cancer clinical trials, patient
  advocate, and cancer research information

Kidney Cancer Association
– www.curekidneycancer.org includes chat room and ask a nurse service.
  http://www.kidneycancerjournal.com/ on-line journal

National Cancer Institute
– http://www.cancer.gov/dictionary/ contains more than 3,500 terms
  related to cancer and medicine.

– www.cancer.gov/drugdictionary drugs and biologic agents currently
  being used in cancer clinical trials are listed in the dictionary which
  provides brief, accurate descriptions of cancer-related drugs and
  biologic agents, including information about chemical class and
  mechanism of action.

– www.clinicaltrials.gov provides regularly updated information
  about federally and privately supported clinical research in human
  volunteers, including information about a trial's purpose, who may
  participate, locations, and phone numbers.

– http://www.medlineplus.gov/ type "renal cell carcinoma" into the
  search box to access twenty-five web links.

– http://www.nci.nih.gov/cancer_information/cancer_type/kidney/
  lists cancer type specific information and clinical trials

NexCura
– www.cancerfacts.com interactive site designed to help patients make
  informed decisions, has excellent descriptions of treatment options.

Oncolink
– www.oncolink.org University of Pennsylvania site that provides
  comprehensive information about specific types of cancer, with
  daily updates on cancer treatments and news about research advances.

People Living with Cancer
– www.plwc.org patient information website of the American Society of Clinical Oncology (ASCO) designed to help patients and families make informed health-care decisions

Physician Orders for Life-Sustaining Treatment Program
– http://www.ohsu.edu/ethics/polst Physician Orders for Life-Sustaining Treatment (POLST) is a one page, two-sided form designed to help health care professionals honor the end-of-life treatment desires of their patients.

Planet Cancer
– www.planetcancer.org provides a unique voice for young adults who have been affected by cancer: fresh and irreverent, but always honest.

Quackwatch
– www.quackwatch.org a nonprofit corporation whose purpose is to combat health-related frauds, myths, fads, and fallacies.

Together Prescription Access
– http://www.togetherrxaccess.com is a free savings program, sponsored by some of the world's largest pharmaceutical companies, that helps qualified individuals and families save approximately 25%-40% on over 275 brand-name prescription drugs and other prescription products, as well save on a wide range of generic drugs.

UroToday
– http://www.urotoday.com provides regularly updated relevant recent news clips, treatment guidelines, clinical trials.

Services

Action to Cure Kidney Cancer
– www.ackc.org a grassroots organization working to raise awareness and to ensure that kidney cancer receives public and private funding.

Abigail Alliance
– www.Abigail-Alliance.org —dedicated to helping gain access to developmental cancer drugs

Angelbus
– www.angelbus.org dedicated to providing compassionate ground transportation for those in need.

Angel Flight America
– www.angelflightamerica.org free air transportation for needy patients
to specialized healthcare facilities. Telephone 1-800-446-1231

Cancer Hope Network
– www.cancerhopenetwork.org offers free one-on-one support.

Corporate Angel Network
– www.corpangelnetwork.org free air transportation for cancer patients
with no financial requirements but you must be able to walk and
travel without life support. Telephone 1-866-328-1313.

National Association of Hospital Hospitality Houses
– www.nahhh.org provides lodging and other supportive services to
patients and their families receiving treatment away from home.
Telephone 1-800-542-9730

National Patient Travel Helpline
– www.patienttravel.org provides information about and referrals to
charitable, long-distance medical air transportation. 1-800-296-1217

Stritter Medical Consulting
– www.strittermed.org provides sliding-fee scale consultation to
meticulously research your case for the latest and best treatments,
discuss it with national experts, and then report back to you in
terms you can understand. 1-650-851-0377

Helpful Questions
This list of questions to ask your physician was compiled by Steve Dunn
and is reprinted from *The Association of Cancer Online Resources*
kidney cancer listserv archives with permission:

Questions re Treatment

1. What is your treatment plan?

2. How many other people have you seen/treated with the same dx as
mine? What are do statistics say about the success rate of the recommended treatment? What is your success rate with cases similar
to mine?

3. Are there any other treatment choices?

4. Present your rationale for the type of treatment which your are recommending.

5. What are the benefits and risks of this treatment?

6. What drugs and dosages will be used?

7. How will the drugs be given and who will perform it?

8. What is the treatment protocol (initial date, time, frequency, duration, etc.)?

9. What are the possible side effects and how should I deal with them?

10. How should I modify my diet during my treatment?

11. Whom should I contact in case there are any complications or if I have any further questions during my treatment?

12. How will the treatment affect my normal activities?

13. I am currently taking the following medicines (vitamins, minerals, herbs). Will this have any effect on the treatment?

14. What are your feelings about the use of complementary approaches (such as: vitamins, minerals, herbs) with conventional treatment? Would you recommend any?

15. What new treatments are being studied in clinical trials?

16. Would a clinical trial be appropriate in my case?

17. If distance travel is involved where will I stay, who will help make those travel arrangements for me? How long can I expect to be away? Can arrangements be made to bring along a caregiver? How much time, travel and expense will be involved and how will it be paid for?

Questions re Follow Up Care

1. What kind of a follow up care do you recommend?
   -nephrectomy - full or partial, regular surgery or laproscopic
   -cystoscopy
   -biopsy
   -urine tests
   -IVP, X-rays, other nuclear tests?
   - MRI, CT Scan, Blood work

   And what are you looking for with each of these tests?

2. What life style changes do I need to make?

3. What signs should I look for to see if my cancer has spread or returned?

4. How often should/will I be followed up on to monitor that I am still cancer free (or that cancer is stable or shrinking is patient is not disease free)?

5. What types of follow up tests will be performed and how often will they be done?

Questions re Second Opinion

1. What are the risks of postponing the treatment in order to obtain a second opinion, and how long can the treatment be postponed without any health hazards?

2. What documentation (test results, reports, etc.) will I need for the second opinion?

3. How can this transfer of documents be arranged?

These are some questions a patient may want to ask the doctor before treatment begins:

What is my diagnosis?

What is the stage of the disease?

What are the treatment choices? Which do you recommend? Why?

What are the chances that the treatment will be successful?

How will we know if the treatment is working?

How long will the treatment last?

How long will the it take to see results from this treatment?

How long will any positive results last from this treatment?

How long will any side effects from this treatment last?

What can I do to take care of myself during treatment?

What new treatments are being studied?

Would a clinical trial be appropriate for me?

What are the risks and possible side effects of each treatment?

How will I feel after the operation?

If I have pain, how can it be controlled?

Will I need more treatment after surgery?

Will I need a skin graft or plastic surgery? Will there be a scar?

Will treatment affect my normal activities? If so, for how long?

How often will I need checkups?

What is the treatment likely to cost?

More questions to discuss with your doctors:

How advanced is the cancer?

Is there a chance of cure or prolonged survival with the treatments suggested?

What are the statistics on general cure rates with this type of treatment?

What is the goal of this treatment?
(Knowing if the goal is cure, prolonged survival, or symptom management will help in evaluating side effects from treatment options)

What is your medical opinion of my case?

What about my social, emotional and financial needs?
(Many patients focus on medical treatment and overlook asking about support for emotional, social and financial issues).

Incidental
Finding

NOTES:

APPENDIX *for* CHAPTER RESOURCES

References for Chapter 5
Towards Effective Therapy:
Cancer Cell Biology and Cancer Research in Renal Cell Carcinoma
— *John A. Copland, Ph.D.*

1. **Jemal A, Murray T, Ward E, et al.** 2005 *Cancer Statistics, 2005.* CA Cancer J Clin 55:10-30
2. **Hanahan D WR** 2000 *The Hallmarks of Cancer.* Cell 100:57-70
3. **Bishop J** 1991 Molecular themes in oncogenesis. Cell 64:235-48
4. **Garbers DL, Dubois SK** 1999 *The Molecular Basis of Hpertension. Annual Review of Biochemistry* 68:127-155
5. **Watson RE, Goodman JI** 2002 *Effects of Phenobarbital on DNA Methylation in GC-Rich Regions of Hepatic DNA from Mice That Exhibit Different Levels of Susceptibility to Liver Tumorigenesis.* Toxicol. Sci. 68:51-58
6. **Morris MR, Gentle D, Abdulrahman M, et al.** 2005 *Tumor Suppressor Activity and Epigenetic Inactivation of Hepatocyte Growth Factor Activator Inhibitor Type 2/SPINT2 in Papillary and Clear Cell Renal Cell Carcinoma.* Cancer Res 65:4598-4606
7. **Hard G** 1998 *Mechanisms of Chemically Induced Renal Carcinogenesis in the Laboratory Rodent.* Toxicol Pathol. 26:104-112
8. **Lock EA HG** 2004 *Chemically Induced Renal Tubule Tumors in the Laboratory Rat and Mouse: Review of the NCI/NTP Database and Categorization of Renal Carcinogens Based on Mechanistic Information.* Crit Rev Toxicol. 34:211-299
9. **Golub TR** 2004 *Toward a Functional Taxonomy of Cancer.* Cancer Cell 6:107-108
10. **Takahashi M, Rhodes DR, Furge KA, et al.** 2001 *Gene Expression Profiling of Clear Cell Renal Cell Carcinoma: Gene Identification and Prognostic Classification. Proceedings of the National Academy of Sciences* 98:9754
11. **Atkins MB, Avigan DE, Bukowski RM, et al.** 2004 *Innovations and Challenges in Renal Cancer: Consensus Statement from the First International Conference.* Clin Cancer Res 10:6277S-6281

12. Copland JA, Luxon BA, Ajani L, et al. 2003 *Genomic Profiling Identifies Alterations in TGF Signaling Through Loss of TGF Receptor Expression in Human Renal Cell Carcinogenesis and Progression.* Oncogene 11:6109-6118
13. Takahashi M, Yang XJ, McWhinney S, et al. 2005 *cDNA Microarray Analysis Assists in Diagnosis of Malignant Intrarenal Pheochromocytoma Originally Masquerading as a Renal Cell Carcinoma.* J Med Genet 42:e48-
14. Tan M-H, Rogers CG, Cooper JT, et al. 2004 *Gene Expression Profiling of Renal Cell Carcinoma.* Clin Cancer Res 10:6315S-6321
15. Yang XJ, Tan M-H, Kim HL, et al. 2005 *A Molecular Classification of Papillary Renal Cell Carcinoma.* Cancer Res 65:5628-5637
16. Kosari F, Parker AS, Kube DM, et al. 2005 *Clear Cell Renal Cell Carcinoma: Gene Expression Analyses Identify a Potential Signature for Tumor Aggressiveness.* Clin Cancer Res 11:5128-5139
17. Kanayama Ho, Lui WO, Takahashi M, et al. 2001 *Association of a Novel Constitutional Translocation t(1q;3q) with Familial Renal Cell Carcinoma.* Journal of Medical Genetics 38:165
18. Serrano M, Massague J 2000 *Networks of Tumor Suppressors. Workshop: Tumor Suppressor Networks.* EMBO Rep. 1:115-119

References for Chapter 7
Renal Cell Carcinoma Epidemiology
— *Alex Parker, Ph.D.*

1. Bergstrom A. Terry P. Lindblad P. Lichtenstein P. Ahlbom A. Feychting M. Wolk A. *Physical Activity and Risk of Renal Cell Cancer. International Journal of Cancer.* 92(1):155-7, 2001.
2. Benichou J. Chow WH. McLaughlin JK. Mandel JS. Fraumeni JF Jr. *Population Attributable Risk of Renal Cell Cancer in Minnesota. American Journal of Epidemiology.* 148(5):424-30, 1998
3. Bjorge T. Tretli S. Engeland A. *Relation of Height and Body Mass Index to Renal Cell Carcinoma in Two Million Norwegian Men and Women. American Journal of Epidemiology.* 160(12):1168-76, 2004
4. Burnet NG. Jefferies SJ. Benson RJ. Hunt DP. Treasure FP. *Years of Life Lost (YLL) From Cancer is an Important Measure of Population Burden—and Should be Considered When Allocating Research Funds.* British Journal of Cancer. 92(2):241-5, 2005
5. Chow WH. Devesa SS. Warren JL. Fraumeni JF Jr. *Rising Incidence of Renal Cell Cancer in the United States.* JAMA. 281(17):1628-31, 1999.

6. Chow WH. Gridley G. Fraumeni JF Jr. Jarvholm B. *Obesity, Hypertension, and the Risk of Kidney Cancer in Men.* New England Journal of Medicine. 343(18):1305-11, 2000

7. Fryzek JP. Poulsen AH. Johnsen SP. McLaughlin JK. Sorensen HT. Friis S. *A Cohort Study of Antihypertensive Treatments and Risk of Renal Cell Cancer.* British Journal of Cancer. 92(7):1302-6, 2005.

8. Hunt JD. van der Hel OL. McMillan GP. Boffetta P. Brennan P. *Renal Cell Carcinoma in Relation to Cigarette Smoking: Meta-Analysis of 24 Studies.* International Journal of Cancer. 114(1):101-8, 2005

9. IARC Monographs, *Tobacco Smoke and Involuntary Smoking,* Volume 83, ISBN 92 832 1283 5, 2004

10. Jemal A, Murray T, Ward E, Samuels A, Tiwari RC, Ghafoor A, Feuer EJ, Thun MJ: *Cancer statistics,* 2005. CA: *A Cancer Journal for Clinicians* 55(1):10-30, 2005.

11. Linehan WM. Vasselli J. Srinivasan R. Walther MM. Merino M. Choyke P. Vocke C. Schmidt L. Isaacs JS. Glenn G. Toro J. Zbar B. Bottaro D. Neckers L. *Genetic Basis of Cancer of the Kidney: Disease-Specific Approaches to Therapy.* Clinical Cancer Research. 10(18 Pt 2):6282S-9S, 2004

12. Lohse CM, Cheville JC: *A Review of Prognostic Pathologic Features and Algorithms for Patients Treated Surgically for Renal Cell Carcinoma.* Clinics in Laboratory Medicine 25(2):433-64, 2005.

13. Mahabir S. Leitzmann MF. Pietinen P. Albanes D. Virtamo J. Taylor PR. *Physical Activity and Renal Cell Cancer Risk in a Cohort of Male Smokers.* International Journal of Cancer. 108(4):600-5, 2004.

14. McLaughlin JK. Chow WH. Mandel JS. Mellemgaard A. McCredie M. Lindblad P. Schlehofer B. Pommer W. Niwa S. Adami HO. *International Renal-Cell Cancer Study. VIII. Role of Diuretics, Other Anti-Hypertensive Medications and Hypertension.* International Journal of Cancer. 63(2): 216-21, 1995

15. McPherson CP. Sellers TA. Potter JD. Bostick RM. Folsom AR. *Reproductive Factors and Risk of Endometrial Cancer. The Iowa Women's Health Study.* American Journal of Epidemiology. 143(12):1195-202, 1996

16. Mellemgaard A. Lindblad P. Schlehofer B. Bergstrom R. Mandel JS. McCredie M. McLaughlin JK. Niwa S. Odaka N. Pommer W. et al. *International Renal-Cell Cancer Study. III. Role of Weight, Height, Physical Activity, and Use of Amphetamines.* International Journal of Cancer. 60(3):350-4, 1995.

17. Menezes RJ. Tomlinson G. Kreiger N. *Physical Activity and Risk of Renal Cell Carcinoma.* International Journal of Cancer. 107(4):642-6, 2003.

18. Moore LE. Wilson RT. Campleman SL. *Lifestyle Factors, Exposures, Genetic Susceptibility, and Renal Cell Cancer Risk: A Review.* Cancer Investigation. 23(3):240-55, 2005.

19. **Murai M. Oya M.** *Renal Cell Carcinoma: Etiology, Incidence and Epidemiology.* Current Opinion in Urology. 14(4):229-33, 2004

20. Nicodemus KK. Sweeney C. Folsom AR. *Evaluation of Dietary, Medical and Lifestyle Risk Factors for Incident Kidney Cancer in Postmenopausal Women.* [Journal Article] International Journal of Cancer. 108(1):115-21, 2004.

21. **Parker AS. Cerhan JR. Lynch CF. Ershow AG. Cantor KP.** *Gender, Alcohol Consumption, and Renal Cell Carcinoma.* American Journal of Epidemiology. 155(5):455-62, 2002

22. **Parker AS. Cerhan JR. Janney CA. Lynch CF. Cantor KP.** *Smoking Cessation and Renal Cell Carcinoma.* Annals of Epidemiology. 13(4):245-51, 2003

23. **Parker AS. Cerhan JR. Lynch CF. Leibovich BC. Cantor KP.** *History of Urinary Tract Infection and Risk of Renal Cell Carcinoma.* American Journal of Epidemiology. 159(1):42-8, 2004.

24. **Ries LAG, Eisner MP, Kosary CL, Hankey BF, Miller BA, Clegg L, Mariotto A, Feuer EJ, Edwards BK (eds).** *SEER Cancer Statistics Review,* 1975-2002, National Cancer Institute. Bethesda, MD, http://seer.cancer.gov/csr/1975-2002/, based on November 2004 SEER data submission, posted to the SEER web site 2005.

25. **Semenza JC. Ziogas A. Largent J. Peel D. Anton-Culver H.** *Gene-Environment Interactions in Renal Cell Carcinoma.* American Journal of Epidemiology. 153(9):851-9, 2001.

26. **Sweeney C. Farrow DC. Schwartz SM. Eaton DL. Checkoway H. Vaughan TL.** *Glutathione S-Transferase M1, T1, and P1 Polymorphisms as Risk Factors for Renal Cell Carcinoma: A Case-Control Study.* Cancer Epidemiology, Biomarkers & Prevention. 9(4):449-54, 2000.

27. **van Dijk BA. Schouten LJ. Kiemeney LA. Goldbohm RA. van den Brandt PA.** *Relation of Height, Body Mass, Energy Intake, and Physical Activity to Risk of Renal Cell Carcinoma: Results From the Netherlands Cohort Study.* American Journal of Epidemiology. 160(12):1159-67, 2004.

28. **Wolk A. Lindblad P. Adami HO.** *Nutrition and Renal Cell Cancer.* Cancer Causes & Control. 7(1):5-18, 1996.

29. **Yu MC. Ross RK.** *Obesity, Hypertension, and Renal Cancer.* New England Journal of Medicine. 344(7):531-2, 2001.

30. **Yuan JM. Castelao JE. Gago-Dominguez M. Ross RK. Yu MC.** *Hypertension, Obesity and Their Medications in Relation to Renal Cell Carcinoma.* British Journal of Cancer. 77(9):1508-13, 1998.

References for Chapter 9
Psychosocial Issues of Renal Cell Carcinoma
— *Steve Ames, Ph.D.*

1. Capuron, L., Ravaud, A., Miller, A. H., & Dantzer, R. (2004). *Baseline Mood and Psychosocial Characteristics of Patients Developing Depressive Symptoms During Interleukin-2 and/or Interferon-Alpha Cancer Therapy.* Brain, Behavior, and Immunity, 18, 205-213.
2. Clark, P. E., Schover, L. R., Uzzo, R. G., Hafez, K. S., Rybicki, L. A., & Novick, A. C. (2001). *Quality of Life and Psychological Adaptation After Surgical Treatment for Localized Renal Cell Carcinoma: Impact of the Amount of Remaining Renal Tissue.* Urology, 57, 252-256.
3. Cohen, L., de Moor, C., Parker, P. A., Amato, R. J. (2002). *Quality of Life in Patients with Metastatic Renal Cell Carcinoma Participating in a Phase I Trial of an Autologous Tumor-Derived Vaccine.* Urologic Oncology, 7, 119-124.
4. de Moor, C., Sterner, J., Hall, M., Warneke, C., Gilani, Z., Amato, R., & Cohen, L. (2002). *A Pilot Study of the Effects of Expressive Writing on Psychological and Behavioral Adjustment in Patients Enrolled in a Phase II Trial of Vaccine Therapy for Metastatic Renal Cell Carcinoma.* Health Psychology, 21, 615-615.
5. Ficarra, V., Novella, G., Sarti, A., Novara, G., Galfano, A., Cavalleri, S., & Artibani, W. (2002). *Psycho-Social Well-Being and General Health Status After Surgical Treatment for Localized Renal Cell Carcinoma.* International Urology and Nephrology, 34, 441-446.
6. Heinzer, H., Mir, T. S., Huland, E., Huland, H. (1999). *Subjective and Objective Prospective, Long-Term Analysis of Quality of Life During Inhaled Interleukin-2 Immunotherapy.* Journal of Clinical Oncology, 17, 3612-3620.
7. Kidd, P. S., & Parshall, M. B. (2000). *Getting the Focus and the Group: Enhancing Analytical Rigor in Focus Group Research.* Qualitative Health Research, 10, 293-308.
8. Krueger, R. A., & Casey, M. A. (2000). *Focus Groups: A Practical Guide for Applied Research* (3rd Ed.). Thousand Oaks, CA: Sage.
9. Stewart, D. W., & Shamdasani, P. N. (1990). *Focus Groups: Theory and Practice.* Newbury Park, CA: Sage.
10. U.S. Department of Health and Human Services. (2004). *The Health Consequences of Smoking: A Report of the Surgeon General.* Atlanta, GA: U.S. Department of Health and Human Services.

Incidental
Finding